20 POUNDS IN 90 DAYS

Kick Food Cravings, Jump-Start Healthy Habits, and Look Great Naked— in 4 Weeks

By Chloe Black

http://www.fitquickapp.com

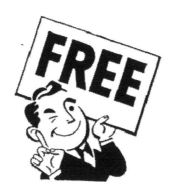

As a show of appreciation to my readers, I've put together FREE motivational resources, including a cheat sheet guide to liquid calories, the "before breakfast" 9-minute exercise routine, and a FREE exercise music playlist.

Click HERE to receive your FREE resources, now!

Table of Contents

Credits & Special Thanks:

Intellitext Transcription Services

Patrick King Consulting

Subversive Photography

Andrea Lynn Tyrell

Katherine Lam

Tara Brite

Jessica Groetsch

Stevonne Ratliff

Mom & Dad

Introduction

My problem? Maybe you have it too.

I *love* food. I love food when I watch TV, before I go to bed, when I wake up, and in restaurants. Mostly I love buttery, sodium packed gourmet 'foodie' food but sometimes, I just want a dirty, crazy, boozy one-night stand with Taco Bell.

As much as I love food, I might love wine even more. What IS food without a nice red Cab to wash it down? Champagne bubbles are a great way to celebrate um, that it's Thursday at 6pm. OR give me a frothy, creamy craft brew any day of the week.

For years, consuming calories was my drug of choice. I honed the art of Yelp.com to be my dealer. Whatever craving I had and whenever I had it, a 20-dollar takeout run would get me my fix.

To makes things more difficult, I worked a sedentary 9-to-5 that required traveling and decadent business meals or just plain airport food junk. I had a tall boyfriend that can eat anything, and I was always finding a way to keep up with him.

When my pants officially stopped fitting, it got harder and harder to blame it on dryer shrinkage. I started to panic a little.

So I tried ALL of the fad diets, including but *not* limited to:

- Juice cleanse (lost 5 pounds of water weight, gained it right back, broke out like I was in middle school)
- Paleo (started eating bacon excessively like some sort of meat candy and developed bizarre fixation with "cheat days" which turned into "cheat weeks")
- Calorie counting (aw -- I forgot to record my calories AGAIN. How many calories is a donut? Like, 70, right?)

- Lemon-Cayenne Cleanse (Great, if you want to spend most of your life in the bathroom)
- All cardio, all the time (I actually GAINED weight. Yeah.)

20 pounds later, to my horror, I have discovered that these extreme weight loss tactics were not working for me.

Which leads me to . . . that feeling.

Maybe you know that feeling. The feeling when the scale doesn't budge for weeks and you throw your hands up in the air and scream, "Starving myself and exercising all the time doesn't make a difference. I'll just eat what I want!"

That's what I did when I couldn't seem to get my weight down, no matter how much I deprived myself of the things I loved.

Maybe you know this feeling too:
- You deny yourself the foods you love only to binge and then feel bad about yourself.
- Food is a potent source of comfort, happiness, and habit.

- You find yourself overdoing it at mealtime, and finish feeling stuffed and full of regrets.
- You may have tried every diet in the book and are familiar with deprivation.
- You just don't have time to workout and get to the gym.
- Gym memberships are costly and just go to waste when busy life gets in the way.
- Your clothes don't fit right and are starting to split because of the weight you've gained.
- Losing weight feels hopeless. You don't even really want to think about it because of so many failed attempts in the past. Instead, you make excuses about big bones, genetics, hormones, or anything to let yourself off the hook for your weight.
- You just want to feel comfortable, sexy, and proud in your own skin.
- You were feeling great until you saw the number on the scale this morning.

Finally, after looking at the scale I realized I didn't have time for any more excuses like 'the holidays' and had to get on the road to being my best self immediately.

I did some serious research and discovered I was eating completely wrong for my body. Not only that, but I was overdoing it on exercise, which was actually causing me to eat more and gain weight.

After this crazy epiphany, I decided to completely reset. I quit processed food and started reading food labels. I put together a super special grocery list and eating plan, and followed it religiously.

Within a matter of months, I had lost 20 pounds and was in the best shape of my life.

Sure, this book is about health. But let's be honest; it's also about feeling sexy. "Sexy" in the that way people who are confident, comfortable, and working to be the best version of themselves are sexy.

In the way that you start feeling like this:

- You wake up every morning feeling great about your body.
- You feel confident and happy when you shop for clothes.
- You eat healthy portions, and know when to stop.
- The food you eat makes you feel nourished and sated.
- Your sex life is now amazing, because you feel comfortable being naked, and are even athletic enough for some exciting new moves.
- Your clothes fit fabulously, except some of them are a little baggy.
- Losing weight feels completely achievable within reach. You are the   master of your own destiny.
- You finally feel comfortable, sexy, and proud of being in your own skin.
- You haven't tried a yo-yo diet in months, your head is clear of the shame, and self-judgment that used to plague your thoughts.
- You've saved a lot of money and grief not jumping on weight-loss trends.

- Food is delicious, but you treat it as fuel that keeps your body running.
- You have finally found way to get regular exercise in your schedule.
- You were feeling great until you saw the number on the scale this morning. Now you feel ecstatic!

The best part is, you won't want to give up after reaching your fitness goals. 20 POUNDS IN 90 DAYS makes sustainable habits a lasting part of your lifestyle so you can reach your healthiest weight and stay there.

If you plateau or miss a deadline, you'll have the tools you need to find a way around it. The 20 | 90 program is designed to work for you for life, forever. Not just until you crash and burn from self-deprivation and jump on the next fad diet wagon.

20 POUNDS IN 90 DAYS draws upon organic, low-carb, low-calorie, and gluten free principles, and is more flexible and forgiving. This means you get to eat carbs and sugar on the program and *still* lose weight. Because who wants to spend the rest of their life without carbs? Not me.

This program is short, to the point, and EFFECTIVE. You will be educated. You will be entertained. But most importantly, you will be kept on track.

And don't get me wrong. I still *love* food. Probably just as much, or more, than you do. That's why I developed this program: so you can be your healthiest, most confident self while still enjoying lots of delicious meals.

Ready? Let's get started.

Chapter 1

Day 1: The Secret to Attraction

You know those people you meet that you just can't take your eyes off of? It's not that they are exotically good-looking; there is just something about them that makes them magnetic.

There is a reason why. Glowing skin, sparkling teeth, healthy hair, and carved abs are all basically just indicators of great health. That is why we find these qualities appealing. We are biologically attracted to healthy people. And the confidence that comes from feeling great doesn't hurt either.

The principle of 20 POUNDS IN 90 DAYS is simple: the healthier your body is, the better you will look and feel. To lose weight and feel fantastic, the best thing you can do is cleanse toxins out of your body. But many people set about doing this the wrong way.

Detoxing does not have to involve shelling out $300 for a trendy juice cleanse, or starving yourself on lemon juice and cayenne pepper for week. Instead, it means consuming food that will restore your body to a natural, healthy state. As modern humans, we already ask our body to process a lot of toxins and allergens from our environment. There is no reason we should be ingesting them in our food.

Every item on the 20 | 90 grocery list contains the nutrient building blocks to a lean body. I'm not exaggerating the list in this chapter is literally comprised of the healthiest food in the world.

Eating these foods will put your body in flawless shape. Losing weight will just be one of the fantastic symptoms that come from eating the most nutrient rich, anti-inflammatory foods available.

The science behind this program is to cleanse your body of toxins and prime it to function on an optimal level. Whether you are trying to recover from an injury, win the world series, get ripped, become bullet proof to allergies, eating these foods can help you achieve all of these things.

The foods in 20 POUNDS IN 90 DAYS have been nutritionist-approved and carefully selected for their micronutrient content, ability to decrease inflammation, attack visceral fat, control blood sugar, boost metabolism, and reduce risk of cancer and heart disease.

These ingredients are also the key to 1,001 recipes, including everything from chicken fajitas to pancakes, so you can satisfy your weirdest cravings.

Oh, and another thing: the 20 POUNDS IN 90 DAYS Grocery List is also surprisingly affordable.

I think you will be pretty thrilled when you find out that whipping up these easy recipes will keep you slim and your bank account fat. So you pretty much don't have any excuses *not* to get started.

Your mission today, should you choose to accept it, is: grocery shop. Your list is below. For the next four weeks and beyond, you should be focused on eating ONLY these foods.

In the next chapter we will dive into something more complex than nutrition, that many diet plans don't usually cover: the science behind human motivation and how you can get prepped with the mental strength you need to jumpstart your habits into the lifestyle you want to lead.

Day 1- Week 1						
1 **Master 90-Day Grocery List**	2 **Introduction** Week 1: Shopping List	3 **Goal Setting** Bacon' Oatmeal, Chicken Salad, BBQ Chicken & Cous Cous	4 **Make It Public** Flaming Chicken Fajitas	5 **Measurements & Before and After Photos** PB&J Buckwheat Waffle, Fancy Clam Pasta	6 **Kitchen Cleanse** Chicken Breast & Asparagus	Week 2- 7 **Weigh-In** Week 2: Shopping List
8 **Vitamin Supplement Regime** Morning Shake	9 **Measuring Food Intake** Cowgirl Chili	10 **Carbohydrates 101** Teriyaki Salmon & Sautéed Garlic Spinach	11 **Fat 101** Skillet Roasted Chicken & Potatoes	12 **Protein 101**	13 **Protein Powder**	Week 3- 14 **Weigh-In** Week 3: Shopping List
15 **Dairy** Cauliflower Vegetable Curry	16 **Sugar** Tomato & Lentil Soup	17 **Budgeting for Healthy Eating** Buckwheat Pancakes with Raspberry Compote	18 **Cardio Exercise** Honey Mustard Chicken & Artichoke	19 **Science of Fat Loss**	20 **Heavy Weights** Swordfish & Spinach Salad	Week 4- 21 **Weigh-In** Week 4: Shopping List, 9-Minute Workout Challenge
Day 22- Week 4 22 **Portion Control & Psychology of Eating** Tomato Tuna Pasta	23 **Snacks & Daily Eating Routine** Apple Crisp	24 **Drinking Calories** Overnight Oats	25 **Hydration** Citrus Sea Scallops, Broccolini, & Faux Mashed Potatoes	26 **Sleep**	27 **Eating Out** Spaghetti Squash with Chicken, Pears, & Parmesan	28 **FINAL Weigh-In Maintenance**

To Sign Up for this Program- Email: info@fitquickapp.com

Grocery List

Here is the master grocery list for the entire program. You should only be eating these foods for the next 90 days. Take it shopping with you, and stick to it.

<u>20 POUNDS IN 90 DAYS Approved Foods List:</u>

Produce (Fruit):

- Lemons
- Limes
- Grapes
- Blueberries
- Raspberries
- Strawberries
- Grapefruit
- Apples
- Cherries
- Peaches
- Pomegranates
- Plums

Produce (Vegetables):

- Lettuce (Red, Green, Arugula, Rocket)
- Frozen and/or fresh spinach
- Artichokes
- Onions
- Asparagus
- Avocado
- Carrots
- Celery
- Cauliflower
- Broccoli
- Zucchini or squash
- Dino kale
- Brussel sprouts
- Bok-Choy
- Pimiento peppers

*Meat

Note: *Whenever possible, meat should be free-range, organic, antibiotic free, and hormone free. Fish should be wild caught from non-polluted ocean regions.*

- Roast chicken (free-range)
- Chicken wings (free-range)
- Buffalo or bison

- Swordfish

- Halibut

- Scallops

- Salmon

- Bacon or pancetta (in moderation)

- Duck

- Hen

- Turkey

- Quail

- Turkey sausage

- Pork

- Venison

- Lamb

Dry Goods, Carbs, and Baking:

- Oatmeal

- Quinoa

- Couscous

- Spelt flour

- Buckwheat flour

- Sliced almonds

- Walnuts

- Dark chocolate

- Coconut sugar or raw, organic brown sugar
- Cacao powder (preferably not processed cocoa powder)
- Kind Bars
- Buckwheat soba noodles
- Barilla Plus pasta

Canned Food:

- Tuna
- Organic tomatoes
- Banana peppers
- Olives
- Anchovies
- Organic, free range chicken or turkey broth
- Vegetable broth
- Beans (kidney, pinto, black, garbanzo)
- Peaches
- Applesauce (sugar free)

Condiments:

- Olive oil
- Coconut oil
- Honey

- Maple syrup
- Vinegar (white wine, apple cider)
- Bragg's Liquid Amino (soy sauce substitute)
- Paul Newman's Oil and Vinegar Dressing (I live on this stuff for salad dressing, marinades, and more)
- Vegenaise (Dairy Free Mayonnaise -- find it at Whole Foods)
- Ketchup
- Mustard (Dijon, spicy brown, and yellow)
- Worcester sauce
- Frank's Red Hot Sauce, Tabasco, or any hot sauce (check ingredients)
- Sunflower Seed Butter (Almond butter works too)
- Sugar-Free Jam (I like blueberry, strawberry, or raspberry)
- Apple Juice -- sugar free (for baking)
- Almond milk
- Green tea

Spices:

- Sea salt
- Pepper

- Garlic powder
- Nutmeg
- Cinnamon
- Vanilla
- Chili powder
- Parsley
- Cilantro
- Basil
- Dill
- Paprika
- Cumin
- Rosemary
- Thyme
- Oregano
- Red pepper flakes
- Curry powder
- Coriander
- Ginger powder

Source: List is extended and adapted from 'The World's Healthiest Foods'

The 'Do Not Eat' List:

- Sugar
- Flour
- Milk
- Cheese
- Butter
- Alcohol (Beer, Liquor)
- Corn
- Soy
- Peanuts
- Sweet potatoes
- Rice
- Anything deep-fried

There are a lot of grey area foods on your grocery list that I don't mention for a reason. This includes eggs, shrimp, eggplant, tomatoes, bananas, and more. If you don't see a food on the grocery list, my advice is to approach cautiously, in moderation. There are excellent reasons they didn't make it into the 20 POUNDS IN 90 DAYS strategy.

For example, shrimp is a great source of protein, but also a cholesterol bombs. With a whopping 152 milligrams of cholesterol per 100-gram serving of shrimp (four or five shrimp), just two servings would put you over the daily-recommended allowance of 300 milligrams.

Tomatoes, eggplant, and peppers are fantastic, colorful veggies loaded with vitamins that can spice up a dish. But these foods are also members of the nightshade family. Nightshade plants present minor autoimmune dangers in the form of chemical compounds called 'alkaloids'. Alkaloids work as a minor 'bug spray' poison, protecting the plant from bugs and molds.

Obviously, we are much larger than bugs and mold, so these plants don't really pose a deadly threat. But the dangers of alkaloids and lectins to humans are gut irritation. Their job in the plant is to kill small things. When introduced to your intestine, the cells lining the intestinal tract are their first victims.

Other foods like bananas and sweet potatoes are generally seen as healthy, but often pack a starchy sugary punch that can derail your healthy eating efforts.

There are enough foods out there for me to write an entire book on each one. If you're curious about this, we will dive into a more science-based exploration of the food nutrient composition in later chapters.

Chapter 2

Day 2: It's All In Your Head

You know those <u>training</u> <u>montages</u> from 1980s movies like Rocky and the Karate Kid? Some inspirational metal music blasts, as you watch the hero grow from a zero to a ripped fighting machine over the course of about 60 seconds.

Well . . . get ready because for the next 28 days, you are going to be the hero starring in your own training montage. And I am going to be your wise and mysterious mentor.

Unlike the 30-second clips in the movies, real-life training montages take 28 days; the time you need to shed your terrible habits like a snakeskin and get seriously addicted to an invigorating new lifestyle.

You already have a book teaching you scientifically tested and proved health information that can turn you into a nutrition genius. Check.

So, here's the hard part. Many people know *how to* exercise and that they *should* eat healthy. But they DON'T! Why not?

Because getting in shape takes will power. And every day life is filled with temptation and distraction (office party cake! movie popcorn!). These little things make our weight loss mission easy to forget or ignore.

For the next 28 days, a lot of the willpower work will be done for you with the recipes and shopping lists in this book. All you need to do is follow the instructions.

Your mission today, should you chose to accept it (and you should), is to shop. That doesn't sound so bad, right?

In the next chapter, I'm going to tell you one of the biggest secrets of weight loss. This part is heavy and hard hitting, because I want you to succeed, and avoid falling into this common trap.

28

WEEK 1: Shopping List

For your convenience, many of the recipes and shopping lists are available online. You can access them by clicking on the link in the title of the recipe.

The password for web page access is: ***healthyhabits***

For every recipe, remember to wash and pat dry raw meat and vegetable ingredients before cooking.

Breakfast

Bacon and Oatmeal

• Steel cut oatmeal

• Maple syrup

• Bacon, ham, or Applegate Farms turkey sausage- check label for sugar

• Almond, cashew, or coconut milk- I prefer this unsweetened Coconut Almond Milk from Califia Farms. Remember to check label for sugar.

PB&J Waffles

• Van's Buckwheat Waffles

• Sugar-free jam

• Sunflower seed butter <u>(cashew or almond butter also works, if budget allows)</u>

Lunch

<u>Roast Chicken Salad</u>

• Extra virgin olive oil for cooking (highest quality you can afford), or double points for avocado oil

• Apple cider vinegar (or balsamic, white wine, or red wine -- your preference)

• Roast chicken (pre-cooked at the store)

• Lettuce (spinach, rocket, or red leaf)

• *Optional toppings: eggs (hard-boiled), sliced almonds, walnuts, pine nuts, avocado, dried cranberries, pepperoncini, salami, or sliced onion*

Dinners

<u>Dinner 1: BBQ Chicken</u>

• 1-2 lb. of chicken drumsticks (double points for organic)

• Ketchup

• <u>Sriracha</u>

• Organic brown sugar

- <u>Bragg's Liquid Aminos</u> or low sodium soy sauce
- Paprika
- Cumin
- Garlic (pre-chopped, or a whole clove)
- Sea salt
- Black pepper

Sides:
- Pearl couscous
- Chicken or vegetable broth (low sodium/ organic for extra points)
- 1 lb. brussel sprouts

Dinner 2: Flaming Chicken Fajitas
- 2-4 chicken breasts (double points for organic)
- 2 bell peppers (your preference of red, green, or yellow)
- 1 Onion (yellow or white)
- 1 Lime
- Avocado (optional)
- Salsa
- <u>Rudi's Spelt Tortillas</u> (found often at Whole Foods) or whole wheat tortillas

Dinner 3: Fancy Clam Pasta

- 2 dozen clams
- Flat leaf (Italian) parsley
- Dry white wine (for cooking, not drinking. Well, maybe a little drinking)
- Crushed red pepper
- Organic soba buckwheat noodles

Dinner 4: Herb Grilled Chicken and Asparagus

- 3-4 organic chicken breasts (6-8 oz. each)
- Fresh thyme
- 2 lemons
- 1/2 lb. asparagus

Dessert

- Berries
- Sugar-free chocolate syrup
- Dark chocolate (extra points for sugar free -- I buy this kind from Trader Joe's)

Chapter 3

Day 3: Put it on Paper

Have you ever wanted to eat healthy and exercise, but just kept putting it off? You know what you're supposed to do and the steps you're supposed to take. But you just don't. You keep saying you'll start tomorrow, or next week, or sometime soon.

Don't delegate all of your weight-loss plans to your future self. That person is no stronger, or better equipped with will power than the person who is reading this sentence right now.

Think about yourself 90 days from now. Don't you want to do that person a huge favor? Imagine waking up in 90 days with the body you want, and a sense of accomplishment that you put in the effort to finally make your life happier and healthier once and for all.

"Someday" is not a day of the week. Whether it's a health problem, clothes that don't fit, allergies, or just watching the scale break new records, most of us need a serious wakeup call from denial to make an impactful life change and let 'someday' become 'today'.

It's time to find your own wakeup call, even if it means spending 24-hours gorging on Jack-In-The-Box and donuts. If one final bender is what you think you need to rid crappy food from your system once and for all, do it. And then never look back. Luckily, I have another powerful mental exercise we can try, so you don't have to go that far.

Most fad diet plans fail because they don't actually address the real hurdle of weight loss: it's all in your head. Set your mind straight, and the rest will follow. Bear with me -- I'm about to get Tony Robbins on you for a second. Getting in shape is actually easier than most people let on, and it feels incredible. Eating healthy and exercising is fun and rewarding. But sometimes in life we're so terrified we won't succeed, we panic and fail before even trying.

I bet the reason you have failed at your resolutions in the past is because your unconscious mind is telling you a story. The story is made up of expectations, beliefs, and perceptions you've developed in your life. And whether or not they're true, you chose to believe them.

You don't realize it now, but this narrative you've created is telling you don't have what it takes to be the happier, fitter, more successful person you want to be. You might have a few other barriers in the way like fear of failure, denial, belief you don't deserve what you want, or just plain food addiction. Thankfully, this is just a narrative and it can be changed and re-written pretty quickly.

Just because you haven't done it in the past, doesn't mean you won't be able to do it in the future. Case study after case study proves that writing down goals, to-do lists, and personal narratives is one of the highest factors leading to success versus failure.

Charles Duhigg illustrates a scientific backed example of this in the book "The Power of Habit". Duhigg describes this finding from a 1992 British study involving lower-class elderly patients

– averaging 68 years old – who were recovering from recent hip or knee replacement surgery.

A psychologist was examining ways to increase the patient's willpower to keep up with the arduous rehabilitation process:

> The Scottish study's participants were the types of people most likely to fail at rehabilitation. The scientist conducting the experiment wanted to see if it was possible to help them harness their willpower. She gave each patient a booklet after their surgeries that detailed their rehab schedule, and in the back were thirteen additional pages--one for each week--with blank spaces and instructions: "My goals for this week are _____? Write down exactly what you are going to do. For example, if you are going to go for a walk this week, write down where and when you are going to walk."
>
> She asked patients to fill in each of those pages with specific plans. Then she compared the recoveries of those who wrote out goals with those of patients who

had received the same booklets, but didn't write anything.

It seems absurd to think that giving people a few pieces of blank paper might make a difference in how quickly they recover from surgery.

But when the researcher visited the patients three months later, she found a striking difference between the two groups. The patients who had written plans in their booklets had started walking almost twice as fast as the ones who had not . . .They were putting on their shoes, doing the laundry, and making themselves meals quicker than the patients who hadn't scribbled out goals ahead of time. The psychologist wanted to understand why. She examined the booklets and discovered that most of the blank pages had been filled in with specific, detailed plans about the most mundane aspects of recovery.

For example, one patient had written, "I will walk to the bus stop tomorrow to meet my wife from work," and then noted what time he would leave, the route he would walk, what he would wear, which coat he would bring if it was raining, and what pills he would take if the pain became too much. In a similar study, another patient wrote a series of very specific schedules regarding the exercises he would do each time he went to the bathroom. A third wrote a minute-by-minute itinerary for walking around the block.

As the psychologist scrutinized the booklets, she saw that many of the plans had something in common: They focused on how patients would handle a specific moment of anticipated pain . . .The patients' plans were built around inflection points when they knew their pain--and thus the temptation to quit--would be strongest.

-Charles Duhigg, The Power of Habit: Why We Do What We Do in Life and Business (p. 144). Random House, Inc. Kindle Edition.

The nurse in this study was surprised to learn that the patients who wrote down their goals healed quickly. But even more interesting, was that if they wrote down their plan of attack in a moment of weakness, this helped them cope and perform far better in moments of being tested.

Recovering from hip or knee replacement surgery is absolutely more painful and difficult than trying to skip donuts for a month. Imagine what you could do if you started writing down your plans to exercise daily and overcome food addiction.

Let's re-write your narrative. Scribbling down how you will handle moments of weakness will skyrocket your mental strength through the roof. When faced with a challenge or moment of self-doubt, you will already have a plan you can refer to that can keep you on track.

Keeping a journal or writing down goals will also force you to reflect on your own inner-critic, see the progress you're making, and bring flawed beliefs or self-doubt into perspective.

So now we know that writing something down, even privately, strengthens your commitment to it. Let's apply that knowledge.

Day Two Mission: Set 2 - 6 Fitness Goals and Write Them Down

Take today to really think about things that have held you back from accomplishing what you want in the past. Write them down, and resolve to get past them. Chose the weight or health level you would like to be at, and write that down too.

Do you want to do a handstand? Fit into an old pair of jeans? Run a 5K? Bench press 200 pounds? Get creative. The more exciting your goals, the more excited you will be to go after them. Then decide that you are going to commit 100% to eating healthy, and working towards these goals for the next 90 days.

Below is your first daily meal plan. Time to get cookin'.

WEEK 1: Shopping List

BREAKFAST 1: Bacon and Oatmeal

Prep time: 4 minutes

Total Cook Time: 15 - 20 minutes

It is important to start your day off with a dose of protein. This will keep your blood sugar steady and keep you from binge eating. Oatmeal and bacon make for a great high-protein breakfast on the go.

To get you into a consistently healthy daily routine, you will be eating these things for breakfast a lot, so keep this recipe handy if you need it.

Oatmeal: Boil 1 cup water. Add ⅓ cup of steel cut oatmeal (none of those instant packets; please read ingredients and make sure it is *just* oatmeal). Bring to a boil and then turn to a simmer for 10 minutes until soft.

For flavor, add ¼ cup almond/coconut milk and 1-2 tablespoons of maple syrup.

Bacon: Fry 1 - 2 strips of bacon in a pan for 15 - 20 minutes until it reaches desired crispness, frequently draining the fat. If you don't have time for that, lay bacon out on a baking pan for 20 minutes at 375 F. Drain the grease and pat dry with a paper towel.

LUNCH 1: 'Chose Your Own Adventure' Chicken Salad

Prep time: 12 - 15 minutes

Total Cook Time: 0 minutes

Buy one of those roast chickens at the grocery store -- extra points for organic.

Slice or break off pieces of the chicken breast and toss it in with the lettuce of your choice (arugula, red leaf, spinach).

The secret to an amazing salad flavor bomb? Spices. Salads often taste boring if they aren't properly seasoned. Toss your lettuce with a generous dose of pepper, garlic powder, extra virgin olive oil, apple cider vinegar, and a pinch of salt.

My salad dressing of choice is <u>Paul Newman's Olive Oil and Vinegar Dressing</u> because it doubles as a great fish and chicken marinade, and doesn't have weird, unhealthy ingredients hiding in it.

For extra intrigue:

<u>Adventure 1:</u> Throw in some nuts (sliced almond, walnuts or pine nuts), avocado, and dried cranberries.

Adventure 2: For a more Italian style, add some pepperoncini, salami, and sliced onion.

DINNER: Brown Sugar Sriracha BBQ Chicken with Pearl Couscous and Citrus Brussel Sprouts

http://fitquickapp.com/resources/bbqchicken/

Prep time: 20 minutes

Total Cook Time: 50 minutes

Ingredients:

- 1 lb. brussel sprouts
- 2 cloves garlic, chopped
- 1-2 lb. of chicken drumsticks (double points for organic)
- 1 cup pearl couscous
- 1.5 vegetable or chicken broth (low sodium/organic for extra points)
- 1/4 tbsp. sea salt
- 1/4 tbsp. black pepper
- 1/4-cup ketchup
- 1-2 teaspoons Sriracha
- 1 tbsp. brown sugar
- 2 tbsp. Bragg's Liquid Aminos or low sodium soy sauce

Brown Sugar Sriracha Chicken:

In a plastic bag, add ¼ cup ketchup, 1-tablespoon brown sugar, 2 tablespoons Soy Sauce (low sodium), and 1-2 teaspoons Sriracha sauce.

Put 1 lbs. (about 6 drumsticks) of organic chicken legs into the bag. Mix chicken around to make sure it covered and let it marinate for anywhere from 15 minutes to 24 hours.

Put the legs on a baking pan and bake at 425 F for 20 - 30 minutes (until juices run clear and meat is no longer pink)

Couscous:

Boil 1 ½ cups chicken broth (low sodium, organic). Then, throw in 1-cup Israeli couscous and turn to simmer for 10 - 15 minutes until soft. Add 1/4 tsp. salt and pepper to taste.

Citrus Brussel Sprouts:

Wash 1 lb. of brussel sprouts, cut them in half, and toss with 2 cloves of dices garlic and 1-2 tablespoons olive oil. Cover them in salt and pepper (about 14 twists of each grinder, or ¼ teaspoon) and put them in the over on a baking tray for 10-15 minutes.

Dessert 1: Berries and Chocolate Syrup

Prep time: 6 minutes

Total Cook Time: 0 minutes

Drizzle some chocolate syrup (sugar free) and balsamic vinegar over berries (blueberries, raspberries, strawberries, or all of the above). Yum!

Chapter 4

Day 4: The Power of Going Public

Now that you've gotten your goals written down, I want you to try one more thing to really obliterate your chances of failure: **tell someone what you are going to accomplish.** Post it on Facebook, call up your mom, do what you have to do.

I have an embarrassing story about the first time I tried this experiment for myself. But first, I have to tell you the fascinating reason why sharing your aspirations with people really works.

Announcing a goal publicly creates social pressure proven to increase your chances of accomplishing your goal 10-fold. There are many studies that prove social commitment really works.

Both Alcoholics Anonymous and Weight Watchers are known for leveraging the value of social accountability for success. These programs provide weekly meetings, and buddies to team up with or sponsors to answer in moments of weakness.

The power of social pressure can be used for good, or evil. As humans, we tend to do everything we can to remain consistent with the public personas we project to other people, even when it means behaving irrationally.

During the Korean War, American soldier hostages were successfully coerced to identify as communists through this subtle but potent strategy. Chinese captors did not use torture or force towards the hostages to persuade them to adopt communist view. Instead, they would innocuously request the men make public commitments to various things. Sometimes the public statements would involve slight praise or agreement with communist principles.

As time went on, the American soldiers began standing by their statements, in an effort to be consistent in their public persona. The need to be consistent with their own declarations eventually led them down a path of collaboration

– without really realizing it. Soon enough, the soldiers began identifying as Red.

Stating your goals to an audience or friend will create a public persona for yourself, that you will start unconsciously living up to. It can also offer clarity on your goals, and keep you accountable for reaching them.

The best part about sharing aspirations? The connection it creates. Something wonderful happens when people hear you are working towards something: they begin to brainstorm ways to help or cheerlead.

I used to skip going public with my goals at all costs because I didn't want to admit to the world and the Internet that I felt, well . . . overweight. But keeping my aspirations private meant I suffered in silence. I was getting absolutely nowhere, moping around all by myself.

So, when I decided to lose twenty pounds in three months, I created an entire Facebook movement dedicated to my efforts. I promised before and after pictures, live on the

Internet, in my underwear glory. You can check out the group here.

Embarrassing? Maybe. But mostly I was surprised by the praise and support I received. Most interesting was discovering how many people had the same goals and insecurities that I experienced.

After that, I was ready to do anything to avoid announcing I blew off my goals to sit on the couch eating potato chips. There is no greater motivation than the humiliation of public failure. I had to follow through.

It worked like a charm. 90 days later, I proudly weighed myself to find I had lost over 20 pounds in less those 3 months, just as promised. Crazy, right? It really works. You can do it too.

WEEK 1: Shopping List

BREAKFAST:

Oatmeal and bacon again! The morning routine is important. You are eating for fuel, not flavor. If you need mix things, cook up some breakfast ham or turkey sausages.

DINNER: Flaming Chicken Fajitas

Prep time: 20 minutes

Total Cook Time: 30 - 40 minutes

Ingredients:

- 1-2 tablespoons olive oil
- 2 tablespoons paprika
- 1-tablespoon cumin
- 1/2-teaspoon salt and pepper
- 1-tablespoon chili powder
- 1-2 tablespoons lemon juice
- 1 tablespoons lime juice
- 1-2 garlic cloves or 2 teaspoons pre-chopped garlic
- 2-4 chicken breasts (double points for Organic)
- 2 bell peppers (red, green, or yellow)
- 1 onion (yellow or white)
- Avocado (optional)
- Salsa

- Rudi's spelt tortillas (found often at Whole Foods) or whole wheat tortillas

1. Cut 2-4 chicken breasts into thin strips.

2. In large bowl, mix chicken with olive oil, lime juice, lemon juice, 2 tablespoons paprika, 2 tablespoons cumin, chili powder, about 4 cloves (or tablespoons) of chopped garlic, and 10 grinds each of salt and pepper.

3. Marinade for 20 minutes while you chop up 1 red bell pepper, 1 yellow bell pepper, 1 onion, and 1 avocado.

4. Grill the chicken for about 10 minutes in a pan, until brown and cooked all the way through. Set aside.

5. Grill the veggies in a pan until soft and browned. Mix in the chicken.

6. Warm up spelt or whole wheat tortillas, and serve with salsa, hot sauce, and avocado slices as a garnish.

Guacamole Optional: Mash-up avocado in a bowl with 1-tablespoon garlic powder, 1/2-cup salsa, 2 tablespoons chopped onion, 2 tablespoons lime juice, and 10-15 grinds of salt and pepper.

Chapter 5

Day 5: Get Off the Hamster Wheel

Let's pretend you're trying to climb a big mountain. But this mountain has no peak. You climb and you climb. You get exhausted and feel like you're going nowhere.

Technically, you're higher than you ever have been, and have made a huge amount of progress, but there with no end goal a sense of satisfaction is always just out of reach. You start getting frustrated and tired, and just want to stop.

When people don't set an end-goal to celebrate, they get trapped on what I call the "hamster wheel" which can lead to exhaustion and forfeit. Or worse, developing fixations and compulsions around weight-loss or muscle-building that are irrational and unhealthy. So for your safety, how do we avoid the climbing the never-ending mountain, or incurring "hamster wheel" syndrome?

"What gets measured, gets managed" - Peter Drucker

Make your goals measurable, and add a deadline. A measurable goal often means assigning a numerical value to your progress. Here's an example of how a goal should be written for maximum effectiveness:

I will lose 15 pounds by July 1st, 2017.

The deadline is the extra kick to keep you focused. Without a deadline to reach the top of your mountain, you might accidentally take a side-trail and get lost. Or if too much time passes, you might forget why you were climbing in the first place.

Remember that the deadline is important, but not life or death. I can't tell you how many times I've set a goal date for myself, and accomplished what I was after just a few days later. It was still gratifying, even if I arrived late, because the view from the top of a goal is always gorgeous. Most importantly, make sure your goals are healthy. You can use a BMI calculator to determine a healthy weight for your height, gender, and age.

54

You can never know how far you've travelled, if you don't know where you started. Let's find out where you are now. With that in mind, you have two missions today:

MISSION #1: <u>Weigh yourself, and measure arms, thighs, waist, chest, and hips.</u>

MISSION #2: Take a Before and After Photo of yourself at your current weight.

Of course, weighing yourself is a great way to see your starting point. But taking body measurements and photos are just as important. Here's why: When we start getting healthy and exercising, we gain muscle weight. Seeing your weight spike, even if it's from healthy muscle mass, can be discouraging and throw you off course. Body measurements can sometimes tell us a lot more about what our body is doing than a scale. Grab a measuring ribbon and weigh and measure yourself every month to stay accountable.

For the first time in history, wearables and health technology make it easier than ever to track and stay accountable for your health. All you need is an iPhone.

The 9-Minute Workout app has a handy feature that allows you to record and track your weight and measurements. Another great way to measure and manage your efforts is to record everything you eat. I swear by the fitness journal app MyFitnessPal. It is truly shocking to be confronted with the truth about how many calories you're consuming.

Before-and-after pictures is another old school technique that is simplified thanks to modern tech. Be sure to snap a selfie at your current weight now, or you'll regret it later. If taking pictures of yourself in your underwear is too daunting at first, instead photograph your scale to remind yourself how far you have come.

Terrifying? Yes. Motivating as hell? You bet.

WEEK 1: Shopping List

BREAKFAST: PB&J Buckwheat Waffle

Toast a Van's Wheat-Free Buckwheat Waffle and spread 1 tablespoon of sugar-free jam and 1 tablespoon of almond seed butter over it. Enjoy with 1-2 turkey breakfast sausages.

DINNER: Fancy Clam Pasta

We're getting' fancy tonight. You might want to invite someone special over to impress. Don't be afraid; if I can cook this, you can definitely cook this.

Prep Time: 15 Minutes
Cook Time: 25 Minutes

Ingredients:

- 2 tablespoons olive oil
- 2-dozen clams
- 1/4 chopped flat leaf (Italian) parsley
- 3 cloves (3 tablespoons) chopped garlic
- 1 cup dry white wine (for cooking, not drinking. Well, maybe a little drinking ;)
- Crushed red pepper
- 1-package organic soba buckwheat noodles
- ¼ teaspoon red pepper
- 1/2-teaspoon (about 14 grinds) sea salt

- 1/2-teaspoon (about 14 grinds) pepper

Chop ¼ cup flat leaf parsley and 3 cloves of garlic. Measure 1 cup of dry white wine. Place ingredients by stove.

Boil pot of hot water. Once it reaches a rolling boil, add package of buckwheat soba noodles to the water. Boil until noodles are soft (but not soggy) and drain. For a taste test, pull out a noodle with a fork, run under cold water, and chew for consistency.

Place large pot or skillet on the stove and warm 2 tablespoons of olive oil on medium heat. Add garlic and stir until it shimmers (30 seconds). Add white wine and 24 clams. Cook 8 minutes until clams open. Discard any that don't open.

Mix the pasta with the clams, wine, and garlic. Add parsley, ¼ teaspoon red pepper, and about 14 grinds of salt and pepper. Mix all together. Buon appetito!

Chapter 6

Day 6: The Simple Trick Steve Jobs Used to Become More
Powerful

I bet you have to make a lot of important choices to make
every day, and some not so important ones, too. Like these:

Organic or not organic?

Do you want a receipt with that?

Fallon or Conan?

Best toilet scrub brand?

Chicken or Beef?

Ugh. Modern life can be exhausting. Just buying toothpaste
from the grocery store involves an overwhelming choice of 20
brands, textures, flavors, and benefits. That is why eccentric
(but brilliant) people like Steve Jobs and John Lasseter decided
wearing the same thing every single day is a good fashion
decision. And they are kind of right.

According to 'The Paradox of Choice', humans have a certain amount of decisions they can make in a day, before suffering from 'decision fatigue'. Decision fatigue means the more decisions you make in a day, the more strain it puts on your willpower, judgment, and ability to control impulses.

The more tiny, not-so-important decisions you eliminate, the more willpower you retain to make earth-shattering decisions when the time calls for it, so you can finally achieve world domination.

Don't waste your limited decision resources constantly trying to decide what to eat. Meal planning in advance, eating the same foods, and establishing a consistent routines are all foolproof strategies to prevent over-thinking your options and staying on course.

Find a few healthy fuel ingredients you love that you can eat over and over again. Keeping these ingredients in my fridge at all times guarantees I am not going to be faced with an emergency hunger situation. If I think 'Maybe I should go grab a bacon cheese burger for lunch' the lazy part of me kicks in and says 'Nahhhh- we already have this roast chicken right here'. Bam! Decision fatigue defeated by ninja kitchen choices.

Limiting food choices will also help you master portion control. In a study performed by food researcher and PhD Brian Wansink, office workers who kept candy in clear dishes on their desks dipped their hand in the bowl a whopping 71 percent more often than those who kept candy out of sight.

When it comes to food, out of sight, out of mind really works. Here is a very simple rule to eating well and maintaining progress: if it's not there, you can't eat it.

Which brings us to today's mission: Go into your pantry and throw away all of the junk. Just clean it out. Maybe even tidy up in there while you're at it. Once you're done throwing out all the garbage, you will have an exciting blank canvas to paint new healthy new ingredients on. While reaching kitchen Zen, remember to compartmentalize all of the different types of food, and keep your options simple.

Protect yourself from making bad decisions in your weakest moments with habit-forming systems. Stocking up on tasty, filling foods will absolutely save you the painful regrets of an accidental one-night stand with a Taco Bell gordita. Your future self thanks you.

WEEK 1: Shopping List

DINNER: Herb-Grilled Chicken and Asparagus

Prep Time: 15 Minutes
Total Time: 25 Minutes

Ingredients:

- 3-4 Tablespoons olive oil
- 2-3 organic chicken breasts (6-8 oz. each)
- 1 Tablespoon fresh thyme leaves (4 sprigs)
- 2-3 organic chicken breasts (6-8 oz. each)
- 1 Tablespoon flat-leaf parsley (optional)
- 1 lemon
- 1/2 lb. asparagus
- 3/4 Teaspoon salt
- 3/4 Teaspoon pepper

1. Heat the oven to 425 F. Wash asparagus, dry, and place on baking pan.

2. Drizzle approx. 1-Tablespoon Olive Oil over Asparagus. Sprinkle or grind ¼ tsp. salt (12 mill grinds) and ¼ tsp. pepper over the veggies.

3. While the oven is heating, chop Up 1 Tablespoon of Flat-leaf Parsley (optional) and pull leaves from the fresh Thyme Sprigs. Set aside.

4. Drizzle ½ tsp. over extra virgin olive oil over the chicken breasts. Season with salt and pepper (about 1/4 tsp. of salt and pepper or 6 turns on a salt/ pepper grinder).

5. Turn the chicken over and repeat so the breasts are coated in oil, salt, and pepper.

6. Put the asparagus in the oven and set a timer for 10 minutes

7. Add 2 tablespoons of olive oil to a pan. Once the olive oil shimmers (after a minute) add the chicken breast and cook for 5-6 minutes on each side. The chicken is done when it's no longer pink in the center.

8. Remove asparagus from the oven and grate lemon rind over it for some added zest. Then slice the lemon into wedges to serve with the chicken.

Voila! You have dinner and lunch leftovers for tomorrow.

Chapter 7

Day 7: 6 Eating Commandments You MUST Follow for Health and Happiness

I hope you had fun getting pumped about your goals. I won't even ask if you told everyone you know that you're doing this program, because I know you already did it. Did you post your goals on Facebook? Great. I can't wait to see your before and after photos.

Let's dive into your eating strategy and break things down into some simple terms. If there is one thing I know, it's this: Proper eating habits are the most important part of getting a leaner, more athletic looking body, hands down. Here are 6 easy to follow eating guidelines Follow them just 80% of the time, you will start losing weight and feeling healthier within a month.

Guideline #1: If You Can't Pronounce It, Don't Eat It (or Just Start Reading Labels)

When we evolved as humans hundreds of years ago, we ate food from the earth that was free of strange things like growth hormones, herbicides, pesticides, artificial sweeteners, trans fat, and other the unnatural things we are exposed to today.

Eat real, whole foods with ingredients you can pronounce. Once you start reading food labels, you will find yourself horrified by the amount of corn syrup, hydrogenated oils, and other poisonous ingredients put in our food to increase the shelf life. It may take some hunting to find a tomato sauce without sugar and corn syrup in it, but it is worth your time.

One great trick to make sure you're buying the right foods: when you enter the grocery store, first walk the whole perimeter with the fresh veggies and, before proceeding to the center aisles.

Guideline #2: The Color Test- Taste the Rainbow

Next time you're about to put something in your mouth, take a second and think:

Is this white? Or is it made with an ingredient that is white?

The more real color food has (inside and out), often the more nutrients it has.

Good Things to Eat:

- Lean meats (i.e. Salmon, Lamb, Buffalo)
- Fruits and vegetables (artichokes, carrots, beets)
- Whole grains (red couscous, black rice, barley, etc.)
- Lentils (chickpeas, kidney beans)
- Spices and condiments for taste (i.e. mustard, paprika, salsa, etc.)
- Healthy fats and oils (i.e. avocados, olives, etc.)

Not So Good Things to Eat:

- White sugar
- Bleached white flour
- Dairy
- Potatoes
- Corn
- White rice

Guideline #3: Start Every Day With a Protein Shake

I am so dead serious about this rule, that when I travel, I pack my blender with me. Maybe you don't have to go that extreme. Eating a little bit of protein when you wake up will go a long way by keeping your blood sugar steady all day.

I take it one step further and pack my morning protein shakes with tons of nutrients that have cleansing benefits. It's pretty much my #1 get-healthy-quick secret. Check out the next chapter for my go-to recipe.

Guideline #4: Avoid Fried Foods

This goes double for foods that are deep-fried or breaded. Braise, boil, steam, bake, grill, roast, sauté, and steam, but don't bread and fry your food. Reheat your food in a pan (not aluminum) instead of the microwave, whenever you can. When grilling or heating your foods in a pan, use safe oils that can handle high temperatures, like avocado or coconut oil.

Guideline #5: Avoid Alcohol, Drugs, and Stimulants

Think of your body like a glass of liquid. Every time you add a toxin to it is like adding liquid to the glass. If you put too many toxins, like a glass filled too full, it will start to spill over. When this "overflow" occurs, your body begins to exhibit reactions to the toxins, in the form of allergies, diseases, health problems, and weight-gain.

Some people think smoking causes weight-loss as an appetite suppressant. This couldn't be further from the truth. It contributes toxins to your body that causes you to bloat and gain weight.

Every element of 20 POUNDS IN 90 DAYS, down the handpicked ingredients, are designed to keep you toxin level as low as possible. For this reason, avoid stimulants altogether, including coffee, salt, alcohol, sugar, soft drinks, cigarettes, and other social drugs.

Alcohol mostly consists of sugar. Even worse, it lowers your inhibitions, causing **you to make bad eating decisions**. Because alcohol is a form of poison, it causes your body to crave food in effort to absorb the alcohol, causing you to overeat. While you're at it, consider quitting fruit juice. Drinking calories (especially drinks with fructose) is pretty much suicide for any serious weight loss attempt.

These types of foods and stimulants cause your blood sugar to spike high and crash like a roller coaster off its tracks, which can lead to hypoglycemia, diabetes, adrenal exhaustion, weight gain, and more.

Now, life is meant to be lived. I get it. If you must pick a poison, go for white or red wine, in a dry varietal like pinot noir or cabernet sauvignon. Wine has the lowest sugar content of all alcohol. If you must drink during this program, try to limit to no more than 2 glasses, twice a week. Which brings me to....

Guideline #6: Forgive Yourself and Have a Safety Plan
Life, and food, is meant to be enjoyed. As long as we're not Cro-Magnons hunting bison and foraging for berries in the wild, eating perfect 100% of the time isn't always possible.

If you find yourself unable to live without some foods, set a 'Cheat Meal' in your calendar, to allow yourself to indulge once a week. Just make sure to exert some extra discipline the rest of the time to maintain a healthy balance.

If you have a moment of weakness, forgive yourself immediately, and keep trying. One mistake won't ruin it all. Don't give up and punish yourself. Just get up and keep going.

WEEK 2: Grocery List (Link)

Password: healthyhabits

Breakfast

- 1-3 grapefruits
- Oatmeal (if you're running low)
- Ham, bacon, or sausage (if you're running low)

Smoothie Ingredients:

- Dino kale
- Frozen blueberries, strawberries, or raspberries

Dinners:

Cowgirl Chili

- 1 lb. ground turkey
- 1-can kidney beans
- 1-can pinto beans
- 2 cans stewed tomatoes (preferably organic, no salt added. Check label for sugar)
- You should already have cumin and paprika from last week
- Cinnamon

- 2-3 white onions

Teriyaki Salmon

- 2-4 pieces wild caught salmon (6 oz. each)
- 100% pure maple syrup (you should already some leftover from last week)
- Bragg's Liquid Aminos or Low Sodium Soy Sauce
- Fresh garlic
- 2 large bunches of spinach or 1 bag (1lb.) frozen spinach

Skillet Roasted Chicken and Potatoes

- 3 chicken thighs (1 lb.)
- 3 drumsticks (3/4 lb.)
- 1 yellow onion
- 2 Yukon Gold potatoes
- Fresh rosemary
- Coriander

Chapter 8

Day 8: The Breakfast Cleanse Cocktail

Good Morning! Rise and shine.

Morning routines are everything. How you start your days often determines how you will spend and finish them. The best thing you can do first thing in the morning is prime your body for mental alertness, healthy digestion, and health.

For years, I've yearned after overly ambitious morning routines, filled with yoga, meditation, and pushups, followed by a healthy, breakfast and productive spurts of work and creativity.

Good luck with that. I'm not an early bird and my mornings are a groggy and panicked dash from bed to bathroom, to closet, to fridge, to front door. Meanwhile, I have managed to find one routine that has transformed my body and eating habits.

This protein shake is one of my favorite recipes to kick start my day. It only takes about 10 minutes to make and gives a morning dose of nutrients that will make you feel energized, full, and steer you away from overeating.

WARNING: This is breakfast smoothie sort of resembles an algae pond. It might taste like it at first too, but trust me; you will learn to love it. And the health benefits are absolutely worth it.

Ingredients:

- **1 scoop whey protein isolate powder**

   Starting your day with a dose of protein will ease your body out of it's nightly fast by regulating your blood sugar and satisfying your body. This prevents you from overeating throughout the day, and primes your body to build lean muscle and lose weight.

   I suggest **Biotics Whey Protein Isolate**, **Tera's Whey Grass Fed Organic Whey Protein, Plain**, OR **Organic**

Plant Protein Powder (for those of you who are hardcore about no dairy or animal products).

- **1 scoop Biotics Nutriclear detox supplement**

  I swear by this stuff. It's a biologically active, hypoallergenic supplement designed to support detoxification and healing in the gastrointestinal tract and liver.

  NutriClear cleanses the body in "metabolic clearing" programs by eliminating the buildup of toxic substances. This enables your body to recover from imbalances, work more efficiently, and ultimately look and feel healthier.

- **1 scoop greens powder.**

  Getting all of your nutrients, greens, and vitamins for the day is a tough feat. Luckily, a scoop of greens powder will make sure you get there. Depending on your budget, I suggest **Purity Products Triple Greens Powder** or **Athletic Greens.**

  http://www.amazon.com/gp/product/B00THEPSPW/ref=as_li_tl?ie=UTF8&camp=1789&creative=390957&cre

- **1-tablespoon organic fresh flax oil.**

  Why flax seed oil? Because of it's healthy dose of
  Omega 3's and polyunsaturated fatty acids (such as
  alpha-linolenic acid). Flaxseed Oil has been known to
  reduce the risk of cancer and heart disease, aid growth
  of healthy hair and nails, and play an essential role in
  burning body fat.

  This healthy form of fat also helps prevent wrinkles. You
  can even rub it on your face to reduce skin
  imperfections, but it is more much effective when
  digested. I could go on all day about how amazing EFAs
  (Essential Fatty Acids) like these are for weight loss,
  health, and disease prevention.

- A few shakes of **cinnamon.**

  Cinnamon is magical- it controls insulin levels, steadies
  blood sugar, Lowers LDL cholesterol, helps burn belly
  fat, and suppresses the appetite. Obviously, you should
  be eating this stuff a lot. Sprinkle some in your morning
  drink.

- 1 hefty squeeze of **lemon juice**– Lemon is an excellent dose of vitamin C (proven to aid weight loss). This not only will add fresh zest to your drink, but also suppress food cravings and work to cleanse your digestive system.

Now for flavor, add your choice of frozen fruits. I prefer:

- **1/2-cup organic frozen peaches, strawberries, blueberries, or raspberries.**
- Brownie points for the Brave: add **1/2 cup of kale** for extra leafy roughage and nutrients.
- **3-4 ice cubes**
- A **splash of water** for easy-blending

Proceed to blend these ingredients into a pulp and drink.

Supplements can be expensive, but considering how much I save on food gorging by drinking this every day, consider the cleansing and nutritional benefits worth it. Your body will be thrilled to get the vitamins it needs and you will be on a much quicker road to your weight loss goal, thanks to the fantastic digestion benefits of this drinks.

Chapter 9

Day 9: Cheat Sheet: Which Diet Trend Should You Be
Following?

For as long as I've been interested in nutrition, I've noticed a
silent war between calorie counters and Paleo diet preachers.
Some people swear by only consuming a caveman diet of
veggies and protein, and others live by tracking their minuit
portions of beer and cheesecake with digital food journals like
'MyFitnessPal'. I have tried both, and guess what? They all can
work, IF you stick to it.

The science of calorie counting assigns a numerical energy
value to the food you consume. If you eat more energy than
you expend in a day, you start gaining weight. For calorie
counting to result in successful weight loss, you must either
eat less or exercise more. To beat the calorie counting game,
you have to measure everything you eat, and make sure your
calories are at a deficit.

Here are a few benefits from counting calories:

1. You might start exercising a lot more, just to enjoy some extra eating perks
2. Eating sweets and carbs in moderation will keep you sane, but over time you will probably start skipping dairy and processed foods to keep your calorie quota in check. This results in an overall healthier eating lifestyle.

I find when I count calories I lose weight slowly, but also keep the weight off longer because my body isn't relying on a state of ketosis to stay trim. It's always a great idea to record what you eat through calorie counting or food journaling just to keep you accountable.

If you just can't find the time to record everything you eat (it's not easy), Paleo might be the method for you. 'Low-carb' diets are a great 'no-brainer' form of calorie counting. Lean proteins and vegetables generally contain a very low caloric dose. When I cut dairy and processed carbohydrates, I naturally find it a struggle to even reach my minimum calorie goal for the day.

Finally, there is a third, more flexible way to monitor what you eat to lose weight. This eating method is called 'macro dieting'. 'Macros' are the three macronutrients that our food is compromised of: protein, carbohydrates, and fat. In the next few chapters, you're going to learn why your body needs all of them.

The philosophy of 'macro' dieting calculates what percentage of your food intake should be dedicated to each macronutrient. With this approach, you don't have to be religiously picky about what types of food you put in your body, and you don't have to count every calorie.

If you would like to try the macronutrient approach, just Google 'macro calculator'. Hundreds of tools will appear in the search results that can help you calculate how many grams of protein and fat you should be consuming each day to reach health or weight loss goals.

WEEK 2: Grocery List (Link)
Password: healthyhabits

http://fitquickapp.com/resources/cowgirl-chili/

Dinner: Cowgirl Chili

This chili will sate you with hearty, delicious protein and healthy carbs for the rest of the week. And it costs maybe 10 bucks to make.

Prep Time: 10 Minutes
Total Time: 50 Minutes

Ingredients:

- 1 lb. ground turkey
- 1-can kidney beans, drained and rinsed
- 1-can pinto beans, drained and rinsed
- 1 can stewed tomatoes (Muir Glen is a great organic brand without sugar in it.)
- ¾ tsp. ground cumin
- ¾ tsp. paprika (optional)
- ½ tsp. cinnamon
- 2 tsps. Chili powder
- 1/3 white onion, diced
- 2 cloves fresh garlic (or 2 tablespoons, pre-chopped or powdered)
- 1/2 tsp. each of salt and pepper

1. Drain and rinse 1 can of pinto beans and 1 can kidney beans. Slice and dice a white onion.

2. Cook a pound of ground turkey in a large skillet over medium heat, piecing it apart with a spatula as it browns. While cooking, add 2 teaspoons chili powder, 1-tablespoon cumin, 1-tablespoon paprika, and 1-teaspoon cinnamon.

3. Once cooked, transfer to ground turkey to large pot and add beans, 2 cups of water, and 2 cans of organics, stewed tomatoes. Bring to a boil, and then reduce heat to simmer for 20 minutes. Add the onion while it's simmering.

4. Enjoy with a Rudi's Spelt Tortilla, warmed on the grill.

Chapter 10

Day 10: The Problem with Paleo

Between fears of high fat, eating red meat, and really any type of carbohydrate, modern eating has become an exercise in insanity. For a while, I read all the contradictory diet science and became paralyzed with irrational food fear. I found myself wandering grocery store aisles with paranoid angst over what to eat, with questions like this echoing in my mind:

- *Should I spend more for organic? What does Organic even mean?*
- *What is trans fat?*
- *Why does everything suddenly have corn syrup and about soybean oil in it?*
- *Should I be eating less carbs? Low-fat? Gluten free?????*

Let's cut through some of the fear mongering to educate you on a few of the food science basics that we as humans, have learned so far. I have no agenda, other than to help you get healthy.

Put on your science cap. Let's sort out some myths and facts of carbohydrates, protein, and fat, and how eating all of them will help you reach your fitness goals.

Everything You Need To Know About Macronutrients: Carbs, Fat, and Protein

The Problem With Paleo

In case you aren't aware of the Atkins craze in the 90's, followed by the recent Paleo explosion, this diet philosophy is based on encouraging you to eat as much food as you want in a day- so long as it is only meat and veggies.

Depending on the fad, sometimes you are allowed dairy, lentils, potatoes, or something else- but never starches like pasta, bread, or grains. The Paleo genre's explosion in popularity has caused an oversimplified view of what constitutes a healthy, human diet.

Most people's take away from Paleo and Low-Carb diets are that ancient humans didn't have access to grains and therefore, this foreign substance is poison to our body.

At first glance, yes, this eating philosophy does share commonalities with what Paleolithic cultures would have eaten, and it does provide a basic strategy for healthy eating. In theory, prehistoric tribes would have done a lot of hunting, fishing, and foraging for plants. That is why grass-fed beef, fish, nuts, seeds, vegetables, and berries are all on the Paleo menu.

Paleo makes the case that modern farming and crop cultivation is what ultimately wreaked havoc on our modern health and lead to obesity. This is why grains and processed flours are forbidden.

Early humans didn't raise animals for meat or milk, so that makes corn-fed animals and dairy off-limits for the caveman diet. And of course, processed foods, refined sugar, and salt as we know it didn't even exist. Our ancestors didn't exactly have Snickers bars and Cheetos 20,000 years ago.

But be careful, because the Paleo diet doesn't take into account the harsh weather conditions or location variances our ancestors dealt with. They absolutely didn't have access to a constant supply of fresh fruits, vegetables, or even bison like we do.

The truth is, while meat and vegetables were a decadent indulgence for ancient tribes, it is likely they spent most of their time foraging and subsisting off of nuts, seeds, grains, and berries.

Their primary protein source? Insects. And some rodents on a good day. So if you really want to commit to eating like a Stone Age purist, you would want to consider whipping up herb-roasted squirrel with a side of grasshopper puree.

The other issue with Paleo is the elimination of grains. Recent finding present that for over 100,000 years humans have been foraging for grains and grinding wheat into bread. Whole grains such as oats and quinoa are not a completely foreign substance to our biological evolution.

And finally, there is no major proof that prehistoric humans enjoyed healthier and longer lives than their modern-day counterparts. Adults were lucky to reach past 40 and most children did not live to adolescence.

A recent study from The Lancet revealed alarmingly high rates of hardened arteries in ancient mummies. 47 of the 137 mummies studied were suspected of having the disease atherosclerosis.

Will you lose weight if you cut out carbs? Absolutely. But it's not because you are embarking on a primal eating quest that will put you in touch with your lost ancestors and ancient self.

It is because eliminating carbs from your diet puts your body into something called 'ketosis'. Put simply, Ketosis is a metabolic process that functions as a backup reserve for your body to keep it going. When you don't have enough carbohydrates for your cells to burn for energy, your body burns fat instead. As part of this process, it makes ketones.

Is ketosis a good thing or a bad thing? Well, it depends. If you're healthy and eating a balanced diet, your body controls how much fat it burns, and you don't normally make or use ketones. But when you cut way back on your calories or carbs, your body will switch to ketosis for energy. Ketosis can become dangerous when ketones build up. High levels lead to dehydration and can alter the chemical balance of your blood. But don't worry- this is rare.

Entering a state of ketosis through fasting or cutting carbs, is a popular weight loss strategy because it burns fat and makes you feel less hungry. It will usually kick in after a few days of eating less than 25 grams of carbs (approximately 3 slices of bread) per day.

Now, Paleo doesn't have it all wrong. It is a high-protein diet, and as you'll soon find out, protein is the basis of all that is pure and good in health. While I don't see anything wrong with ketosis-based diets,I personally have never found 'no carbs ever' to be a sustainable, long-term weight loss plan. It's just too extreme. I wind up binging on bacon to distract myself from thinking about cake cravings. Then I start taking cheat meals, which turn into cheat days, which turn into cheat weeks.

It's all much simpler to start the day off with healthy bowl of oatmeal in the morning, to ward off bad-carb cravings throughout the day.

On occasion, ketosis is a powerful secret weapon that is nice to keep in your tool belt. It can work wonders if you need to drop those last few stubborn pounds, or get ripped quickly for a big event.

In these situations, I go on a 'carb cleanse' for a limited amount of time (3-6 weeks). If you would like to experiment with a 'carb cleanse' to boost your efforts, you can follow the meals I send you, but skip the breakfast oatmeal and replace whole grain side dishes with lentils (pinto beans, chickpeas, or hummus).

If the idea of never eating another tortilla or bowl of fettuccine again in your life terrifies you, I encourage you to learn how to incorporate healthy, complex carbs into your eating habits from the start. I can show you how.

The Case for Carbs

Carbs have gotten a bad rap. The truth is, some are good for you, and some are bad. Of course, if you process anything beyond recognition, it reaches a point where it just isn't healthy anymore.

This doesn't mean carbs are to blame for the obesity epidemic--it just means that eating processed foods loaded with sugar makes people fat. Basic forms of carbohydrates include fiber, starches, and sugar. Carbohydrates are made up of sugar molecules, which your body breaks down into fuel, especially when you're performing intense exercise.

"Carbs" are also found in most foods, from apples to spinach. So no one can actually cut all carbs from their diet, and keep living to brag about it. Your body needs carbs, because without them, your body will begin to break down your muscle tissue to fuel your body. This will sabotage all of your weight loss efforts entirely.

There are three types of carbs:

Simple Carbohydrates
Simple carbs include white sugar, candy, cake, beer, soda, macaroni, and cookies. Most of the time, these carbs should be avoided, aside from occasional indulgences. These are the "bad carbs" that everyone is raging against.

Complex Carbohydrates

Complex carbs include everything from oatmeal, quinoa, bulgur, apples, peas, and cardboard. Just kidding about the last one.

Your body takes both complex and simple carbohydrates and tries to break them down into useable sugar energy to fuel your muscles and organs. It's not the type of carbohydrate that really matters, but how quickly your body can break it down, and how much your blood glucose levels spike during this process.

To calculate carbohydrate quality, there is a more sophisticated method called the glycemic index (GI). The GI classifies foods by how high they boost blood sugar levels, and quickly your body is able to process them.

This philosophy revolves around eating food that are minimally processed and carbohydrates that digest slowly. This means enjoying whole barley or bulgur instead of Wonder Bread and donuts. This type of approach is often easier to stick to, because it doesn't try to entirely eliminate any of the important macronutrients (like fat or carbohydrates) from your diet.

Complex carbohydrates are great because they stabilize your metabolism and blood sugar, which keeps you feeling fuller, longer. They also give your body the energy it needs to perform vigorous workouts. With the GI diet principles, you can have your cake and eat it too, as long as the cake is made of buckwheat.

Last but not least, are **fibrous carbs**. This includes foods like green veggies, lettuce, cabbage, broccoli, sprouts, spinach, cauliflower, peppers, cucumbers, and zucchini.

Neither quitting carbs forever nor consuming a ton of whole grains is the secret answer to weight loss. It is still important to eat proper portions of healthy foods that fuel your metabolism and keep your body's engine running clean.

WEEK 2: Grocery List (Link)
Password: healthyhabits

BREAKFAST:
The Breakfast Salad Smoothie
Turkey Sausage or Bacon

½ Grapefruit

DINNER: Teriyaki Salmon and Sautéed Garlic Spinach

Prep Time: 10 Minutes

Total Time: 30 Minutes

Ingredients:

- 2-4 pieces wild caught salmon (6 oz. each)- *If salmon is out of season, buy frozen and thaw, or sub with chicken breast*
- 1/4 cups 100% pure maple syrup
- 1 tablespoon Bragg's Liquid Aminos or Low Sodium Soy Sauce
- 5 cloves fresh garlic (I keep a jar of pre-diced garlic on hand for emergencies. This will also work.)
- 2 large bunches of spinach or 1 bag (1 lb.) frozen spinach

1. Heat oven to 400F.

2. Smash, peel, and dice 5 garlic cloves.

3. In a glass-baking pan, add 2 tablespoons maple syrup, 1-tablespoon Bragg's Aminos or low-sodium soy sauce, 1-2 garlic cloves, and ½ tsp. salt and pepper to taste.

4. Stir in salmon with mixture, making sure it is fully coated. Marinate for 20 minutes in fridge (if you have the time).

5. Put salmon in oven, and set timer for 20 minutes. Check the salmon at the 16-minute mark to see if it is light pink with a flakey texture. If yes, take out to cool. If not, cook a few more minutes.

6. While the salmon is cooking, heat 2 tablespoons olive oil (or avocado oil) over medium heat until it shimmers. Add 2-3 cloves of garlic to the oil.

I like to leave the garlic in, but you can also remove it from pan after about a minute, once the olive oil is fully flavored.

7. Add the fresh spinach to the pan, slowly adding more as the spinach wilts down.

Or, if you're using frozen spinach, add all of it and break it into smaller pieces with your spatula as it thaws.

---

8. Cook for 2-3 minutes as spinach wilts down or until frozen spinach is full thawed. Mix in ¼ tsp. salt and pepper to taste.

9. Remove salmon from the oven and serve with spinach.

Chapter 11

Day 11: Fat: Luke Skywalker or Darth Vader?

Fats: Luke Skywalker or Darth Vader?

The era from the 1950's to the 1980's was a weird time when a lot of strange food myths started being perpetuated. During this time, we decided animal fat like butter and bacon grease was bad for us.

This is partly because of the irrational logic that eating fat would cause your body to *become* fat. This misconception seems to have spawned some of the worst food trends that exist today. Let's tear a few of them apart.

Before carbs became the scapegoat, fats were blamed for every health problem under the sun. For nearly twenty years, people assumed "low-fat" was synonymous for "healthy".

This caused a lot of food companies to water down fatty ingredients in food, and replace them with sugar for flavor, all so they could plaster a 'low-fat' sticker on the label.

But according to CDC data, when our nation's fat consumption decreased, obesity rates began to skyrocket. Many factors are thought to have contributed to the rise of obesity during this time. Specifically, a spike occurred in the size and frequency of meals, as well as the consumption of sugar.

This makes sense; because we now know that eating healthy fats make us feel full. So when we started eating less fat, we began eating more food. And when we replaced fat with sugar for flavor, our sugar intake went up.

Fat is a critical component of your diet and chances are, you aren't getting enough of it. Fat is proven to be healthy for your heart, muscles, and testosterone levels. Not only that, it is a critical coating for your nerves.

The coating provided by fat speeds up conduction down the nerve so that neurochemical signals are sent through your body efficiently. Put simply, your brain uses fat to tell your body to do things faster.

Research suggests that about 20 to 35 percent of your daily calories should come from fats. Here's what you should know about the different types of fats, and how you can eat more of them.

Monounsaturated Fat

Monounsaturated fats are wonderful, because they have been shown to fight weight gain, lower bad-cholesterol, raise good-cholesterol, and reduce body fat levels. You can find this type of fat in delicious foods like pistachios, almonds, walnuts, and cashews, and high-fat fruits like avocados.

Polyunsaturated Fat

In case you've ever wondered why people, especially body-builders, get really excited about fish oil, this is your chance to find out.

Polyunsaturated fats are special because they contain important omega-3 and omega-6 fatty acids, which are oftentimes referred to as essential fatty acids (EFAs).

These fatty acids cannot be created by our bodies, and have been mostly been processed out of our food. Studies suggest that EFAs protect against type 2 diabetes, Alzheimer's, age-related brain decline, heart disease, and bad cholesterol.

For this reason, it is absolutely crucial you find a way to include these fats in your daily food intake. That is why I spiked your morning detox drink with flax seed oil. You're welcome.

You can also find polyunsaturated fats in fatty fish such as salmon, mackerel, and tuna, as well as from walnuts, flaxseed, sunflower oil, and sunflower seeds.

Saturated Fat

Foods containing high proportions of saturated fat include animal fat products such as cream, cheese, butter, whole milk, and fatty meats. Saturated fats are pretty controversial. Just to clear things up for you, *saturated fat is no longer associated with heart disease.*

Saturated fats are some of the most sating foods, meaning they keep you fuller longer. Research shows diets that are high in saturated fats are often lower in total calorie consumption. In fact, saturated fat is how your body gets its energy. This is why we naturally store carbohydrates as saturated fat.

Certain vegetable products also have high saturated fat content, such as coconut oil and palm kernel oil. You can also find saturated fat in prepared food like dairy desserts and sausage.

The Exception: Trans Fat

Another strange thing happened when people decided fat was bad: we decided to turn vegetable oil into a solid to be used a butter substitute. Food manufacturers thought because it was 'vegetable oil', trans-fat was still healthy, and the food industry was excited because it had a longer shelf life than butter.

Trans fats are made by a chemical process called "partial hydrogenation". This is the chemical that occurs when liquid vegetable oil, a healthy monounsaturated fat, is packed with hydrogen atoms, and converted into a solid fat. This solid has a high melting point and smooth texture, which is perfect for being re-used in deep fat frying.

But the 1990s, the evidence became clear: When vegetable oil is turned into a solid, it still acts like butter inside the body. Trans-fats raise low-density lipoprotein (LDL) or "bad" cholesterol levels. This contributes to the buildup of fatty plaque in arteries. Consuming high amounts of trans-fats has been correlated to increased risk of heart attacks and diabetes, among other terrible health problems.

So, in our misguided effort to eliminate fat from our diets, we happened to create the most poisonous fat of all time, one that is far more dangerous than bacon or cream will ever be.

I don't like to villanize any kind of food. But let's face it: trans-fat is basically Darth Vader of the nutrition world. This is because trans-fat isn't really food, but a man-made chemical. If you are serious about your health, or the idea of eating plastic grosses you out, avoid trans fats as much as possible.

In case you want to watch out for them, trans-fats are often found in French fries, non-dairy creamer, margarine, potato chips, fast food, and anything deep-fried. If food is pre-packaged, you can probably bet is has its share of trans fats. It is also a good idea to stay weary of pre-packaged cake mix, doughnuts, microwave popcorn, and refrigerated dough.

WEEK 2: Grocery List (Link)

Password: healthyhabits

BREAKFAST:

The Breakfast Salad Shake

Turkey sausage, ham, or bacon

½ grapefruit

LUNCH: Teriyaki salmon and spinach leftovers

DINNER: 1-Skillet Layered Roasted Potatoes and Chicken

This is a tasty and complete meal, all cooked in 1 skillet so you can save time and cut out the hassle of dishes.

Prep Time: 15-20 minutes

Cook Time: 1 Hour

Ingredients:

- 1 yellow onion
- 1/2-cup water
- 2-3 Yukon Gold potatoes
- 1-tablespoon olive oil
- 2 tablespoons fresh rosemary leaves (2 Sprigs)
- 1.5 tsp. sea salt
- 3/4 tsp. ground black pepper
- 1-tablespoon coriander
- 4 small, bone-in chicken thighs (1.25 lbs.)
- 4 chicken drumsticks (1 lb.)

Layer 1: Thinly slice a yellow onion, and cover an oven-safe skillet with layers of the slices. Pour a half-cup of water over the onion.

Layer 2: Wash and slice 2 potatoes (with skins) into ¼ inch slices. Layer them over the onions. Drizzle with oil.

Layer 3: Cover with 2 sprigs of fresh rosemary, pulled from the stem.
Add 14 grinds of both salt and pepper.

5. In a bowl, put a tablespoon of coriander and about 24 grinds of salt and pepper. Add 4 chicken thighs (1 and 1/4 lbs.). Rub the spices all over the chicken with your fingers.

6. Lay the chicken skin side up, over the potatoes.

7. Roast the chicken at 425F for about an hour, until potatoes are tender and chicken is no longer pink

Chapter 12

Day 12: Nutrition's Golden Child

Protein is the golden child of nutrition, and never really seems to stir up much controversy. Protein repairs damaged bone, skin, teeth, and hair, and spares muscle mass. Protein also helps create an anabolic hormonal environment (good for muscle building and fat loss), and provides a lot of the materials you need to build your muscles.

You can enjoy protein without worrying about health problems because there aren't any. My favorite thing about protein is this: the more protein you eat the more calories you burn. This is because it is one of the most metabolic macronutrients around.

Don't forget calories are still calories. You can't go on a crazy protein bender and eat as much as you want. The optimal daily protein consumption is about 1 gram per pound of goal body weight.

Your body can't make protein on its own by combining other nutrients, so you have to make protein a priority to achieve the healthiest body possible.

There are two categories of protein: complete and incomplete. Protein is comprised of smaller molecules called 'amino acids'. There are twenty-two amino acids that warrant attention. Our body can manufacture 13 of these amino acids on their own, but for the other nine, it needs our help.

The nine amino acids that we get from food are called "essential amino acids". A **complete protein** is one that contains adequate portions of the following nine amino acids: Tryptophan, Lysine, Methionine, Phenylalanine, Threonine, Valine, Leucine, Histidine, and Isoleucine.

These amino acids also help your body create hormones that help regulate things like blood pressure and blood sugar levels, which are directly responsible for your metabolic rate and muscular growth. An **incomplete protein** lacks one or more of these amino acids. The complete proteins you need are found in foods such as fish, poultry, eggs, and red meat.

Chapter 13

Day 13:What Would Cheech and Chong Drink?

So now that we know why protein is the darling of the diet world: because it promotes lean muscle growth, fat loss, cardiovascular health, and a healthy metabolism.

Suddenly it makes sense whey protein shakes and powders have exploded onto the supplement scene. If you are pursuing a vegan or vegetarian lifestyle, ramping up your workout routines, or recovering from an injury, protein powder is key to optimizing your muscle recovery and growth.

There are thousands of different brands and types, from soy to whey to vegetable protein. So, in case you ever find yourself confused in the supplement aisle, here is a quick crash course of what you need to know.

The Difference Between Protein Concentrate and Isolate:

Protein concentrate is created when the non-protein parts are removed from various high-protein food sources (whey, peas, rice, soy, and more). The result is a powder that's 70 to 85 percent pure protein. The remaining 15 to 30 percent still consists of carbohydrates and fat.

"Isolation" takes this process one step further, and removes a higher percentage of non-protein content. The additional processing creates a premium protein that is up to 95 percent pure. This is why I prescribe whey protein isolate in the morning Detox Cocktail.

Whey Protein vs. Casein

Remember little Miss Muffet who sat on her tuffet, eating her curds and whey? Whey is a byproduct that comes from the process of turning milk into cheese. Whey is also quickly absorbed by the body, making it useful for post-workout recovery.

Casein is another type of dairy protein, produced using a separation process applied to liquid milk that can concentrate milk protein from carbs and fats. We are going to learn lots of interesting and disturbing things about casein in another chapter, but for now, here are the basics.

The main difference between casein and whey protein powder, is the release process. Casein digests over a long period of time, whereas the body rapidly absorbs Whey protein.

That means whey powder is perfect to drink first thing in the morning, or right after a workout when your body is screaming "FEED ME". Casein should be consumed right before bed, to give your body a dose of protein it can keep slowly snacking on all night.

There is also egg protein, made by separating out yolks and dehydrating the egg whites. Egg protein is rich in vitamins and minerals, but eggs are also a common allergen that many people struggle with. Because both casein and whey are dairy-based proteins, the sugar found in milk (lactose) is also common allergen that can make these powders indigestible for some.

If you cannot live with eating animal byproducts, or have intolerance to egg and dairy, you have some other options to explore. Other plant proteins include pea and rice protein, which are hypoallergenic. This means they are easily digestible and almost entirely used by the body, not relieved as waste. However, both pea and rice protein are also deficient in some amino acids, and therefore should not be your primary source of protein.

Hemp and soy are one of the few plant protein sources that are complete proteins, and offer all of the essential amino acids. Soybeans are thought to have a range of benefits from improving immune function and bone health, to reducing the risk of certain cancers and cardiovascular disease.

However, because soy is cheap, most diets are already rife with it, to the point of overexposure. If you start reading food labels, you will quickly notice soybean oil is in nearly everything. Soy has also come under heavy scrutiny lately, due to its effects on hormone levels and estrogen.

Last but not least is hemp protein, which would definitely be the first supplement choice for Cheech and Chong. Derived from the seeds of the cannabis plant, hemp includes all 21 amino acids, is vegan-friendly, extremely hypoallergenic, and a "super food" source of essential fatty acids.

Because cannabis is still a controversial plant to grow, hemp protein is more expensive and difficult to come by than whey. However, it is the superior option if you are looking for the perfect vegan plant protein. Far out, man.

Chapter 14

Day 14: How to Lose 5 Pounds In a Week

You know what's the worst? Being patient. Going to the DMV, sitting at red lights. Heavily anticipating the chiseled 6-pack you've been working so hard for. If your sacrifice isn't balanced with some kind of reward (feeling great about your newly rockin' body) you become seriously vulnerable to quitting before your strategy has a chance to work it's magic.

In other words: **discouragement happens.** Discouragement IS THE ENEMY. It has destroyed many of my most admirable fitness attempts. Here are some sounds of discouragement:

My gym membership is over-priced. I miss doughnuts. Why doesn't my stomach resemble a cheese grater yet?

And that's when the excuses start.

My body is just naturally this weight- nothing changes it. I might as well eat whatever I want and skip the gym.

BAM. Your lazy, sloppy eating habits take over your positive attitude like weeds.

But what if I told you; you could melt 5 pounds off your frame by being an impatient quitter? That's right. I'm telling you to quit.

The quitting strategies below will give you the boost of instant gratification you need to lose weight, and ward off that little devil of discouragement on your shoulder.

1. Quit alcohol

The weight loss I experienced from quitting alcohol for a month blew my mind. Turns out a 'beer gut' is not just for the heavy drinker. Within two weeks of quitting my 'glass of red wine a day' habit, I had lost 10 pounds and deflated like a popped balloon. My jeans fit better and my smile sparkled more. Life was also much more fun without a lousy hangover.

2. Quit dairy

You know those murder mystery movies where you don't know who the killer is until the end of the movie? And it turns out to be a lovable character your were certainly sure was innocent?

Well that is what happened with dairy and I. I thought we were buddies. I loved my mozzarella balls. I put special Trader Joe's goat chèvre on everything.
And then I started counting calories. I quickly realized dairy is just a calorie grenade waiting to obliterate all chances of weight-loss success.

Quitting dairy put me in the best shape of my life, and forced me to examine the high-allergenic properties it had in my diet. The tragic perils of dairy are coming up in another chapter. This is need-to-know information so hang tight.

3. Quit sugar

Despite the deceptively sweet taste and colorful packaging, processed sugar is basically the enemy of all that is pure and good. It's a tough addiction to quit, but if you can pull it off, I commend you. You will be rewarded greatly with energy and health. And yes, you'll quickly shed pounds too.

Are you ready to accept the quitter challenge? It takes 30 days to feel the full benefits of quitting these things, so consider sticking with it. The extra boost will give you the motivation you need to keep going, or help you hurdle over a tricky weight-loss plateau.

WEEK 3: Grocery List

Breakfast/ Dessert:

- Buckwheat flour (extra points for certified gluten-free)
- Baking soda
- 1 large banana
- 6 or 12 pack of large eggs (organic, cage free)
- Vanilla extract
- Blueberries or raspberries (at least 2½ cups)
- Optional: arrowroot powder
- Unsweetened almond milk
- Cinnamon
- Coconut or brown sugar

Dinners:

Exotic Cauliflower Vegetable Curry:

- Vegetable or chicken broth (you'll need at least 5 cups this week)
- Celery stalks (also great for snacks)
- 2-4 medium carrots (also great for snacks)
- 1 can red or yellow lentils
- Tomato paste
- 1 bay leaf
- Ground Cumin
- Ground Coriander

Tomato and Lentil Comfort Soup

- 1 sweet potato
- 1-bag cauliflower florets (will also be great for snacks)
- 2 yellow onions
- Curry powder
- 2 (15-ounce) can chickpeas (garbanzo beans), rinsed and drained
- 2 (14.5-ounce) cans low sodium diced tomatoes, undrained
- Fresh cilantro

Tangy Honey-Dijon Chicken

- 12-24 ounces uncooked Boneless, Skinless Chicken Breasts
- 2 lemons (for juice and zest)

- Honey (¼ cup)

- Mustard (¼ cup - preferably stone ground)

- 1 tablespoon Parsley, fresh chopped

- Dried basil (1 tablespoon)

- Smoked paprika (1 teaspoon)

- Sea salt and pepper, to taste

- Garlic powder

Sides:

- Artichoke

- Vegenaise (can be found at Whole Foods)

- Low-sodium soy sauce or Bragg's Aminos

- Red quinoa (optional)

- Chicken or vegetable broth (optional)

Swordfish Steaks with Purple Moon Dijon Spinach Salad

- Swordfish (6-12 ounces) or chicken if you're on a budget

- Paul Newman's Oil and Vinegar (if available)

- Garlic (chopped or fresh)

- Olive oil or avocado oil

- Salt and pepper

- 5 cups fresh spinach

- 1/2-cup walnuts (optional)

- 2 red onions

- Apple cider vinegar

- Dijon mustard

- Honey

Snacks (Optional, to your preference)

- Hummus

- Sunflower seeds or almonds

- Raspberries or strawberries

- Pre-roast chicken (store bought, extra points for organic)

- 1 medium avocado

Chapter 15

Day 15: Your Brain on Dairy

I want to tell you a story about one of those moments in my life when everything I thought I knew, changed. I'll never forget it. I had been working out several hours a day, every day, and gaining weight. I couldn't figure out what was wrong.

At this time, one of my main food groups was mozzarella. I thought because cheese was both vegetarian and Atkins approved, it must be some sort of protein rich food of the gods.

Looking back makes me chuckle at my young self. So sweet. so naïve. Thankfully, I went to a nutritionist and paid $300 to get some good information, that I'm now going to tell you now, for much cheaper.

Here's the thing: I don't like to flat out tell people that dairy might be the problem with their diet. I can't tell people this, because most of the world's population is literally cracked out on cheese. It's like telling a drug addict they shouldn't do drugs. Doesn't go over great.

I'm not exaggerating. You love cheese so much, because there is morphine in it. Yep, that same drug given in hospitals for hardcore pain relief.

Not only that, but milk provokes similar effects to opiates thanks to the protein casein, which becomes more concentrated in cheese. For this reason, cheese has actually been termed "dairy crack".

So if you're eating cheese, it's not actually the flavor you're into. You love cheese because you're actually into dosing yourself with a little bit of opium and morphine.

Did you know 60% of adults are lactose-intolerant? The ability to digest milk is actually a genetic mutation. That's means there is a 3 in 5 chance you're lactose intolerant. OR you're an X-Man, dairy-tolerant mutant.

I, myself, AM a weird mutant and am not lactose intolerant. But I still avoid milk because I feel suspicious of corn and hormone diet that cattle are fed, and that inevitably wind up in their body secretions. Another reason I avoid milk and dairy is that it contains lactose, which is by definition, a sugar. Dairy is also ridiculously high in calories.

Once I realized dairy was pretty much the ultimate culprit in all of my weight-loss goals, I quit it for six months and never looked back. After cheese rehab, I nearly forgot the stuff existed. I not only lost a ton of weight, and also all interest in dairy.

Cheese addiction is a personal choice every person has to make for him or herself. But I wanted to make sure you are armed with the knowledge that it's probably better to consume cheese, milk, and butter in moderation.

If you must partake in dairy, here are some healthy forms of that may have enough nutrients to justify their existence in your diet:

- Pasture-raised (grass-fed) full fat butter and cream.
- Aged cheeses made from pasture-raised milk. European cheeses are generally grass-fed and aged cheeses are generally more digestible than non-aged cheeses, because they have already partially broken down by microbes.
- Yogurt - unsweetened, plain, or plain Greek.
- Kefir - fermented (cultured) milk with 2-10x more probiotics than most yogurts. Kefir is the healthiest, most digestible form of dairy available and is known to heal many digestive problems (7 - 50 Billion probiotics per cup).
- Lassi - another form of fermented milk, Indian style, and similar to Kefir.

Unhealthy Forms of Dairy:
- Homogenized/pasteurized commercial milk - homogenized milk fat is thought to be harmful to health due to the microscopic fat particles that are formed from the homogenization processing.
- Processed non-aged cheeses such as American cheese or cheese spreads
- Skim milk or fat-free dairy of any type

- Yogurt that is loaded with sugar or artificial sweeteners (most brands)

Now, if you're worried about the calcium you might miss out on from cutting dairy, all you have to do is add more spinach to your diet.

BREAKFAST:

Morning Protein Shake

Oatmeal with Coconut/ Almond Milk, Maple Syrup, and Cinnamon

Ham Slice or Turkey Sausage Link

DINNER: Cauliflower Vegetable Curry

Ingredients:

- 1 1/2 teaspoons olive oil
- 1 cup diced peeled sweet potato
- 1-cup small cauliflower florets
- 1/4 cup thinly sliced yellow onion
- 2 teaspoons curry powder
- 1/2-cup vegetable broth

- 1/4-teaspoon salt
- 1 15-oz. can chickpeas (garbanzo beans), rinsed and drained
- 1 (14.5-ounce) can low sodium diced tomatoes, undrained
- 2 tablespoons chopped fresh cilantro

Directions:

1. Heat olive oil in a large nonstick skillet over medium-high heat.
2. Add sweet potato to pan; sauté 3 minutes. Decrease heat to medium.
3. Add cauliflower, onion, and curry powder; cook 1 minute, stirring mixture constantly.
4. Add broth, salt, chickpeas and diced tomatoes and bring to a boil.
5. Cover, reduce heat, and simmer 10 minutes or until vegetables are tender, stirring occasionally.
6. Sprinkle with cilantro and serve

Chapter 16

Day 16: 10 Hidden Sugar Bombs Ticking in Your Kitchen

Cutting out sugar is trendy right now -- Tom Hanks and Alec Baldwin are <u>supposedly</u> doing it, and for good reason. In 1822, it took the average American *5 days to consume the amount of sugar in a single 12-ounce can of soda* (40 to 48 grams). That is slightly more than 2 teaspoons of sugar a day. Today, we eat 10 to 12 teaspoons every 7 hours (33 teaspoons a day, or 550 calories.)

Our bodies do need small amounts of the sweet stuff, but we get more than enough from natural sugars in almost everything we eat, like oranges or pasta. Maple syrup and honey are also natural forms of sugar, but sugar nonetheless.

'Added' sugar is the white processed crystals we are most familiar with. This is the stuff you associate with lollipops, cookies, and Coca-Cola. Fancy words for added sugar include corn syrup, evaporated cane juice, and almost anything with ending with 'ose'.

As pure white and innocent as it may look, it is sweet, sweet poison. Excessive sugar just as addictive than smoking, and is not much better for you either. So it makes sense that food brands would leverage our sugar addiction by spiking everything from tomato sauce to salads.

Evidence shows a sugary diet does cause cavities and weight gain. But the recent correlation between sugar and heart disease is terrifying. A 15-year study from JAMA Internal Medicine followed participants whose sugar intake was 25% or more of their daily calorie intake. These subjects over twice as likely to die from heart disease than those whose diets contained less than 10% added sugar. The more sugar they ate, the more the risk for heart disease increased.

Sugar is hard on our bodies because it contains fructose, which can only be processed by our livers a little bit at a time. Too much fructose overloads the liver, causing sugar to turn into fat.

You can try to go all out and eat nothing with sugar in it. There are many <u>programs out there that offer sugar addiction</u> rehab. I'm 100% for eliminating sugar from your diet. But dang- is it tough. If you're thinking of quitting sugar, you should know, it's like the Kardashians on TMZ: EVERYWHERE. Trying to quit sugar can require similar mental focus as running for president or climbing Everest.

While going cold turkey is a great idea, you can make huge strides just by cutting hidden sugars from your diet. Sugar bombs disguised as innocuous foods are lurking in every grocery store aisle. Dodging these bullets will make more room in your diet to enjoy a taste of something that *should* be sweet, like apple pie.

1. Yogurt

Yogurt is considered a 'health' food, which is why it can wreak such havoc. People unknowingly consuming gobs of sugary flavored yogurt, thinking it's a healthy.

Skip flavored Yoplait and opt-in to full-fat, plain Greek Yogurt. You can add your own delicious flavoring like nuts, vanilla, cinnamon, or sugar-free jam. Plain yogurt also makes an incredible sour cream substitute for potatoes or chili.

2. Ketchup and BBQ sauce

These foods compliment salty meat dishes so well because they're packed with sugar. Consider whipping up your own condiments at home, or just squeeze mustard on your burger instead.

3. Flavored oatmeal

Flavored packages of oatmeal almost always have 'evaporated cane juice' somewhere in the ingredient label. Prepare your own 'on the go' oatmeal by separating it into ziplock bags to carry around with you, or making a large batch early in the week and adding hot water to reheat. You can season it with Greek yogurt, almond milk, nuts, or dried fruit.

4. Almond and soymilk

Any 'milk' substitute du jour is potential sugar land mine. Remember to grab the 'unsweetened' bottle off the shelf, and check for added sugar.

5. Pasta Sauce, canned tomatoes, and ketchup

128

Tomatoes are already a sweet fruit, which is why it's strange that nearly every canned tomato product in the grocery aisle is exploding with added sugar. Jars of pasta sauce can have as much sugar as a pop tart. Be sure to read the label first, or whip up your own recipe at home.

6. Canned fruit, dried fruit, and applesauce

A lot of canned fruit is soaking in syrup. Apples are already rich in natural sugars, so unsweetened brands like Santa Cruz Applesauce will taste just as delicious, but without the corn syrup.

7. Jam and fruit preserves

This can be an easy one to avoid with a quick glance at the label. Jam is delicious without sugar, and the sugar-free stuff will be easy to find.

8. Bottled tea and fruit juice

I dare you to find a beverage at a gas station (aside from water and Diet Coke) that doesn't contain ten times the amount of recommended daily sugar intake. So-called 'health' drinks and teas from Arizona, Snapple, and SoBe are brimming with the sweet stuff. Chug at your own risk.

9. Pre-packaged meals

This category includes frozen pizza, microwave dinners, soups, and even chili. If someone else has prepared a store-bought meal for you, it probably means a little extra sugar or salt has been thrown in for flavor. Preparing meals and recipes at home is the only real way to truly protection from unnecessary sweeteners.

10. Salad Dressings

The salad dressing and condiment aisle at the grocery store is a veritable nightmare of extraneous sweeteners. After excessive label reading, I can confidently say Paul Newman's Oil and Vinegar is the only dressing I feel safe drizzling on my lettuce. You can also just whip up your own salad topping with a little oil, vinegar, and spices. Be sure to swap sugary balsamic for apple cider vinegar.

I know this chapter was a little scary. Again, no food is evil or off-limits. Everything in moderation. Sugar will find it's way into your diet some way or another, but it is better if you are aware and in control of when it does. Both sugar and dairy are served best as an occasional spice, instead of a major food group.

BREAKFAST:

Morning protein shake

Oatmeal with coconut/ almond milk, maple syrup, and cinnamon

Ham slice or turkey sausage link

DINNER: Tomato and Lentil Soup

Feel free to pair this with one of the chicken dishes from earlier in the program, if you're looking for extra protein.

Prep Time: 20 Minutes

Total Time: 40 Minutes

Ingredients:

- 1-tablespoon olive oil
- 1 medium onion, chopped
- 1 garlic clove, chopped
- 2 celery stalks, chopped
- 2 medium carrots, chopped

- 1-teaspoon ground cumin
- 1-teaspoon ground coriander
- 3/4-cup red or yellow lentils
- 1-tablespoon tomato paste
- 3 cups vegetable stock (certified gluten-free if necessary)
- 2 cups water
- 1 (14 ounce) can chopped or diced tomatoes
- 1 bay leaf
- Salt and pepper, to taste

1. Chop up the garlic, carrot, celery and onion. Prep and set aside ingredients above.

2. Heat oil in pan over medium high, add onion, garlic, celery, carrots and stir until softened.

3. Stir in cumin and coriander and add lentils and tomato paste. Mix in stock, water, tomatoes, bay leaf, and season with salt and pepper.

4. Bring to a boil, then reduce to medium-low and cover with slightly with lid, cooking 15-20 minutes until lentils are soft.

5. With a blender, puree soup until smooth. Adjust salt and pepper to taste.

Chapter 17

Day 17: Why Whole Foods is Wrong

How to Save Money by Eating Healthy

Today I want to address an important question: Is eating healthy expensive?

Despite what Whole Foods has led us all to believe, NO. Eating healthy is not just for privileged and royalty.

You will find that if you follow these grocery lists and recipes in this course, you will eat out less and actually save money. Here are five visible ways eating better will cut your grocery bill in half:

1. Protein powder

Investing in a high-quality protein powder for approximately $30 will provide you with one meal a day for a whole month, which winds up costing about $1 a meal.

2. Oatmeal

A 28-ounce can of oatmeal or porridge costs less that $5, and can provide you breakfast for almost two months. That is less than 20 cents per breakfast.

3. Buying frozen and in-season food

This may surprise you: frozen fruits and vegetables are often healthier than fresh fruits and veggies. It's because they are packaged and frozen in season, the second they are plucked from the ground.

The fruits and vegetables in grocery store aisles are often shipped from other countries, covered in chemicals to keep them fresh, and are about a month old by the time they reach you. This is another great reason to wash and clean your foods properly.

Buying fruit, veggies, and fish that is currently in season will help you eat locally to avoid chemicals, and save you money.

4. Spices

It's important to invest in basic pantry items and spices to make your healthy food taste delightful. Consider it a necessary, upfront cost that will save you money over time. Purchasing spices allows you to make simple, low-cost foods taste exceptional and gourmet.

5. Food addiction

When I eat healthier, I also eat in moderation because I'm not shelling out cash for my next edible fix. Losing your appetite for salty, over-buttered restaurant food will spare you tons of cash every month.

Now, even if it does cost you a little extra to eat healthy, you need to consider this: *life isn't as enjoyable for unhealthy people.* Think about it: there is really no better investment you can make than taking care of your own body. Leading a healthier lifestyle is proven to boost your mood and increase your quality of life.

You will be happier. You will live longer. And generally, people will like you more. Because people like being around happy, healthy, confident people. That alone is worth an extra investment of $100 or so a month.

Your mission today: treat yo' self! Go buy a top-shelf, fancy item that is really healthy for you. This could be some cacao cashew milk, top-of-the-line extra virgin olive oil, a jar of almond butter, you decide. Go crazy and have fun.

BREAKFAST: Banana Buckwheat Pancakes and Berry Compote

Pancake Recipe

- 1 1/2 cup buckwheat flour (certified gluten-free if necessary)
- 1-teaspoon baking soda
- 2 teaspoons cinnamon
- 1 large banana, mashed
- 2 large eggs
- 1-teaspoon vanilla extract
- 1/2 cup unsweetened almond milk (or milk of choice)

Berry Compote

- 1 1/2 cups fresh or frozen blueberries or raspberries
- 1/2-tablespoon coconut (or granulated) sugar

- 1/2-teaspoon vanilla extract
- 1/2-tablespoon water
- Optional: 1/2-teaspoon arrowroot powder (to thicken)

Directions:

1. Preheat a large skillet over medium-low heat.

2. In a large mixing bowl, whisk together all of the pancake ingredients until you have a smooth batter.

3. Grease the skillet with butter or coconut oil, and use a 1/4-cup measuring cup to scoop the batter onto the skillet. Cook the pancakes for 2-3 minutes on the first side, then flip and cook for another 2 minutes. Continue with the rest of the batter.

4. To make the blueberry compote, combine the berries, coconut sugar and vanilla in a small saucepan over medium heat.

5. Use a wooden spoon to stir until the sugar coats the berries. Gently break up the berries with the spoon until they start to

break down and turn into a thick sauce. If it is not as thick as you would like, you can add about a teaspoon of arrowroot or tapioca starch to the sauce. Stir to thicken.

6. Top pancakes with compote sauce and enjoy!

Chapter 18

Day 18: The ONE Thing That Will Make You Smarter +
Cut Your Chance of Disease in Half

Think about your life 20, 40 or 60 years. Would rather be a high-functioning senior badass who makes dorky puns and plays with your grandkids? Or would you rather be a drooling potato in a nursing home?

There is one single habit you can develop that will make the difference in your quality of life. And that habit is **aerobic exercise.** Getting your heart pumping just twice a week halves your risk of general dementia. It cuts your risk of Alzheimer's by 60 percent.

Exercise not only makes you more attractive and healthier, it also makes you smarter. According to John Medina, author of 'Brain Rules', experiments show exercise positively affects executive function, spatial tasks, reaction times and quantitative skills.

It is true that if you wants spent all day sitting around noshing on celery sticks, you would eventually wither away into a weak pile of nothing. But it would take a really long time. Why not reach your fitness goals in twice the time, with an incredible daily exercise strategy? We better get started. Here is the plan:

Rule 1: Break a sweat every single day

For this, the FitQuick app will be essential. I chose this app because it progresses in difficulty and length, as you get stronger. I've included a 9-Minute Exercise routine for you in Chapter 21; to make sure you get the daily dose of aerobic exercise you need, now.

It is great because you can do it anywhere, with no equipment or gym, so you can't fall off the wagon when you're busy or traveling. You can also repeat or lengthen the exercise duration to get a full 30-minute or hour.

Rule 2: Exercise 1 hour, 3-5 x Weekly

In order to see results, you must do some real cardio or strength training for an hour, at least 3 times a week. If hardcore exercise sounds like a little much for you, just start with a 30-minute daily walk to burn off 100 calories.

There also no need to overexert yourself and spend hours at the gym. Exercising beyond an hour can exhaust your body and be counter-productive for weight-loss. Allow yourself to rest to recover at least one day a week.

Rule 3: Have Fun With It

Enjoying exercise will keep you going back. Mixing up your routine will keep you challenged and in better shape. Look up some local gyms in your neighborhood. Try yoga, Bar Method, or start a boot camp. Who knows? Maybe karate is your thing. Most gyms offer a free trial so you have nothing to lose.

Today's Mission: Break a Sweat

Seriously, walk out of your house right now and make some beads of sweat drip from your forehead. Take a jog. Do kick squats. Clean your kitchen. Jump on the latest Zumba craze. I don't care what you do, or how you do it. Just go for it. If you're really lacking ideas, keep reading for an exercise routine I swear by.

BREAKFAST:

Morning Shake

Buckwheat pancake with PB&J

DINNER: Baked Honey Mustard Chicken

Prep Time: 15-20 Minutes

Total Time: 60 Minutes

You Need:

- 24 ounces uncooked boneless, skinless chicken breasts
- ¼ cup honey
- ¼ cup mustard (preferably stone ground)
- 1-tablespoon parsley, fresh chopped
- 1 tablespoon dried basil
- 1 teaspoon smoked paprika
- 1-tablespoon fresh lemon juice
- Sea salt and pepper, to taste

- 1 large artichoke

- Veganaise (you can find this dairy-free mayo at Whole Foods)
- Low-sodium soy sauce or Bragg's Aminos
- Red quinoa (optional)
- Chicken or vegetable broth

1. With a sharp knife, slice off the top of the artichoke, and the stem of the artichoke. Use scissors to trim off the sharp part of artichoke leaves.

2. Rinse the artichoke, and place it in a large pot of water to boil for about 20 minutes, until leaves can be picked off easily.

3. Bring 2 cups of vegetable or chicken broth to a boil. Then add 1 cup of quinoa. Bring to a boil and let simmer for 15-20 minutes until soft. Season to taste with salt and pepper.

While the artichoke is boiling- get started on the chicken:
1. Preheat oven to 375 Fahrenheit.
2. Rinse and pat dry chicken breasts and place in a large glass dish. 3. Season them with sea salt and pepper.

4. In a small bowl, stir together the remaining ingredients (spices, mustard, and honey) and pour over the chicken. Flip each one over a few times to coat it well.

5. Place on a metal cooking tray. Cook for 45-50 minutes in the oven, turning and basting them half way through.

Handy Tip: You can always make sure the chicken breasts are fully cooked by inserting a meat thermometer into the thickest part of the breast to assure an internal temperature of at least 165 degrees Fahrenheit. If you don't have a meat thermometer, slice into the thickest part of the breast to assure there is no pink.

Yum! Your food is now ready. Dig in.

Chapter 19

Day 19: When You Lose Fat, Where Does It Go?

Have you ever lost weight, and wondered...where did it go? Does it go to the Bahamas? Or outer space? Is it off to a Twilight Zone dimension where all lost things go- like half pairs of socks and missing car keys?

This media misinformation surrounding fat loss these days also adds more confusion to this question. For example, The New York Times likes to post inflammatory headlines claiming that exercise isn't the way to lose weight. While the article goes on to basically contradict itself, it is unclear if they are actually waging a war against cardio, or just trying to create Internet scandal.

But even NY Times can't deny- there are thousands of reasons why you should workout: it helps you live longer, increases your quality of life, makes you happier and smarter, and prevents disease. Plus, it just feels good to get stronger and kick butt. But yes, exercise also helps you lose weight. And there is some fascinating biochemistry to prove it.

Many people think that fat is processed as food and excreted as waste, or that it converts to muscle. But this is wrong. Mass can't be created or destroyed, so the atoms that make up your triglycerides have to go somewhere.

To "burn off", fat must go through a complex biochemical process. Scientist Ruben Meerman put this question to the test, and came up with the scientific equation for what happens to fat once it "gets lost".

Here is a very broad equation to sum-up Meerman's study: $C_{55}H_{104}O_6 + 78O_2 \longrightarrow 55CO_2 + 52H_2O + energy$.

In simplified terms, this equation means that when you metabolize fat, you end up with carbon dioxide, water, and energy. So how do we lose fat? By exhaling it.

According to Meerman, 84% of the fat you burn will be exhaled into the atmosphere as CO_2, while 16% of the mass will transform into H_2O. Your fat will ultimately go to feed plants, while the other small amount of water you lose will be expended through sweat, urine, or other bodily fluids.

Exhaling CO_2 will help you lose weight -- and exercising is the healthy way to exhale more. For this reason, the traditional approach of eating less and exercising more will inevitably get you to your weight loss goals.

In the next few chapters, you will find a simple exercise routine to help you start breathing heavy, along with some special mind tricks to help you master the art of portion control.

Chapter 20

Day 20: How to Burn Calories While Napping

A lot of people believe that if they lift heavy weights they will 'bulk up' like Mr. Universe. But this is a women's magazine myth. Lifting weights is actually great for women aiming to look slim and curvaceous. Whether you are man, woman, or bunny, the best way to transform your body and increase muscle tone is to incorporate heavy weights into your workout routine.

The reason? Muscle tissue is the number one factor impacting our metabolism, above meal frequency, hydration, and even genetics. Muscles are live tissues that burn calories through the regeneration process.

The more muscle you have, the more calories you burn, regardless of age or activity level. Lifting heavy weights will help you burn more calories during your workout and can even increase resting metabolism by 8 percent.

That's right. When you lift heavy weights, you can burn calories just by taking a nap. That 8 percent can add up to more than 5 pounds a year.

Another study from the University of Alabama in Birmingham showed that dieters who lifted heavy weights lost the same amount of weight as dieters who did just cardio, but all the weight lost by the weight lifters was primarily fat while the cardio camp lost a lot of muscle along with some fat.

So how can you take advantage of this exciting new knowledge? Next time you go to the gym, instead of doing 20 repetitions of bicep curls with a 5-pound weight; try doing 5 reps with a 20-pound weight. Or when you do lunges or squats, grab a heavy weight to add an extra challenge.

When experimenting with strength training, it is important to go slowly and focus on perfecting your form. To prevent injury, be sure to consult with a trainer or take a class that can teach you how to lift properly.

The best part? Fewer repetitions with heavier weights will cut your workout time in half. And if getting "big and bulky," is your fear, you can rest easy knowing pumping it in the weight room will only fight off fat.

DINNER: Swordfish Steaks with Red Couscous and Purple Moon Dijon Spinach

Saladhttps://drive.google.com/file/d/0B2Wjg5CN0sbFLWdp WmZNYWV0cU0/view?usp=sharing

BREAKFAST:

Morning Protein Shake

Bacon and Eggs

DINNER: Swordfish Steaks and Purple Moon Dijon Spinach Salad

Prep Time: 15 Minutes

Cook Time: Total Time: 25-30 Minutes

Swordfish Steaks:

These delicious steaks are tasty, scrumptious, and worth the price! But do feel free to sub this meal out with a chicken recipe if you're on a budget.

1. Mix 2 tablespoons Paul Newman's Oil and Vinegar, 1-2 tablespoons lemon juice, 1 tablespoons garlic (powder or fresh chopped), 1-tablespoon parsley, and 1/2 tsp. salt and pepper to taste.

2. Add Swordfish Steaks and coat with mixture entirely. Put steaks in the fridge and let marinate up to 20 minutes (if you have time). In the meantime, mix the salad dressing.

3. Heat olive or avocado oil in pan on MEDIUM-HIGH until oil faintly smokes; add fish. Cook swordfish for 3-4 minutes on each side. You will know it' cooked when the fish has turned white all the way through, and is slightly browned on the outside.

Purple Moon Dijon Spinach Salad:

Wash and dry the spinach and set aside. Chop a red onion into halves (until they look like moon shapes).

In a medium saucepan, add 1 tablespoon olive or avocado oil with 2 tablespoons apple cider vinegar, 2 tablespoons Dijon mustard, and 1 tablespoon honey. Add 1/4-tablespoon salt and pepper to taste.

Add the purple onions to the to the pan, and let cook until soft (but still slightly crispy). Pour the sauce and onions over the spinach and toss until it the spinach is slightly wilted. Optional: Add walnuts or bacon bits for an extra crisp.

Chapter 21

Day 21: The 9-Minute Workout Challenge

For a visual demonstration of this routine, go to
FitQuickApp.com.

9-MINUTE WORKOUT CHALLENGE

Do each of the 9 Exercises below for 45 seconds, with a 15
second break in between.

1. **Side to Sides**

1. For this Cardio Warm-up, start stranding in a neutral
position with feet hip width apart and toes facing forward
2. Jump to your left, and lift your right foot off the ground
slightly and bending your knees into a slight squat
3. Shuffle to your right side, lifting up your left leg. Repeat this
motion from side to side.

Bonus Challenge: Place an object of 10 inches or so on the
ground (you can also tape a line on the ground and pretend
there is an object). With your knees bent and upper body
looking forward, jump over the object from one side to the
other at a fast pace.

2. Roll-Up Jumps

Muscles Worked: Gluts, Hamstrings, Quads, Abs, and Lower Back.

1. Stand with feet hips width apart and squat down, slowly lowering your seat and then back onto the mat.

2. Roll all the ways back so that knees are overhead, and then roll forward and up to standing.

3. Right away do a quick jump while reaching your hands up high towards the ceiling.

4. After landing, squat down to the floor and repeat the move.

Bonus Challenge: Do a tuck jump (instead of just a jump) at the end. Jump up and tuck your knees quickly into your chest, before coming down to the ground.

Do: Keep your abs tight throughout this exercise

3. Fire Hydrant

Muscles Worked: Gluts, Abs

1. Place your body on an all-fours position. Elbows should be slightly bent.

2. Back should be parallel to the ground, not arched or swayed downward. Hold abs tight and keep a flat back.

3. Keeping the kneeling position raise left leg out to the side, parallel to the ground. Maintain for a second and slowly return to the initial position.

4. Repeat movement with same leg until set is finished. Repeat the exercise using the right leg.

Bonus Challenge: Place a 5-pound weight under your knee and squeeze tight as you complete your set.

Don't:

- Force or swing the leg raising motion.

- Raise leg any higher than a horizontal level position.

- Arch the lower back--keep back flat and abs strong.

- Allow the knee with the working leg touch floor.

Do:

- Take the exercise slow to feel the burn

4. Hollow Body to Boat

Muscles Worked: Core Strength, Abs

1. Lie down flat on back and push belly button down towards the floor, your lower back should be touching the ground
2. Keep your abs and butt tight at all times, and with your arms pointed straight overhead and legs straight with toes pointed
3. Start slowly raising your legs and shoulders off the ground
4. Your head should come off the ground along with your shoulders, with your ears are glued between your shoulders
5. Slowly bend your knees, bringing them into your chest, while thrusting your arms straightforward, so you are balancing on your seat
7.Alternate from Hollow Body position to Abs Boat for one repetition. Repeat.

Do:
- Keep your lower back rounded and on the ground
- Keep your abs and seat tight the entire exercise
- Start with your arms and legs higher (1-2 feet high off the ground) and slowly build up strength until they can be held lower (just inches off the ground) without breaking the position.

Don't:
156

- Let your back arch

- Touch your feet or hands to the ground

5. Jump Rope/ Line Jumps

1. Bounce your feet off the ground in rapid succession.

2. Think about keeping your torso erect, standing tall, keeping your abdominals tight and staying light on your feet.

6. Modified Push-ups

Muscles Worked: Chest, Triceps, Shoulders, Abs, and Gluts

1. Begin by getting down on yours hands and knees with your hands just outside shoulder width and slightly forward of your shoulders. Your knees should be directly aligned with your hips. Keep your abdomen tight and your spine in a neutral position.

2. Bend your elbows and lower chest to 90 degrees at the elbows. Keep your palms flat on the floor for the entire exercise.

3. Slowly exhale, keep your abs tight and your seat tucked in. Hold the position for the length of the set, keeping your head, back, and hips aligned.

Bonus Challenge: If these are easy for you, try full push-ups with feet on the ground, instead of knees. Place your hands on a bench, chair or step as long as it is stable and secure to take your body weight.

Don't:
Don't let your hips sag to the ground.

Do:
Tuck in your seat and squeeze your gluts.

7. Elevated Triceps Dip

Muscles Worked: Triceps, Abs, and Shoulders

1. Place hands shoulder width apart, fingers facing forward and elbows pointing backwards with a slight bend in the elbows.
2. Place feet on the ground and legs extended out in front of you with a slight bend in the knee.
3. Lower yourself until your elbows are bent to about 90 degrees. Then press back up to straight arms.

Optional: Place your hands on a bench, chair or step as long as it is stable and secure to take your body weight.

Bonus Challenge: Kick your right or left leg straight and off the ground, alternating straight leg every 30 seconds.

Do:

- Keep your chest up and your back straight at all times

Don't:

- Lock your elbows
- Drop your head
- Shrug your shoulders. Keep them down and away from your ears.

8. Knee Ups

1. Stand in a neutral position, and place your hands palm down in front of your waist
2. Bring your right leg up so that it touches your right palm
3. Quickly lower your right leg, and bring the left leg up to hit your left palm. Kick your bent legs up, alternating in rapid succession to hit your palm each time.

Do:

- Pretended like you are giving your upper legs a high five with your hands

- Alternate legs quickly so you are almost jogging in place

- Challenge yourself by lifting your legs up high to reach your hands

9. Bicycle

Muscles Worked: Core Strength, Abs

1. Lie on your back with knees bent, feet on the floor, and hands behind your head (don't clasp your fingers).

2. Press your lower back into the mat and tighten your ab muscles

3. Lift your head, shoulders, and upper back off the floor and simultaneously move your right elbow and left knee toward each other while straightening your right leg (don't let it touch the ground).

4. Draw your right knee back up and immediately move your left elbow and right knee toward each other while straightening your left leg; that's one rep.

5. Continue to move continuously, as if pedaling a bicycle.

Do:

- Keep your abs tight, and you lower back on the ground

- Open your elbows

___

- Try to shoulder to your opposite side knee while doing the crunch

Don't:
- Cave your neck and elbows in

And- that's it! Nine minutes of HIIT exercise. Congratulations. You've completed your exercise routine for the day.

Now it's time to do some shopping. It's week four and you're in the final stretch!

<u>WEEK 4: Grocery List</u>

Breakfast:
- 2 medium bananas
- 1/3-cup oats (certified gluten-free if necessary)
- Greek yogurt (small container)
- Pecans (1 tablespoon)
- Unsweetened almond milk
- Chia seeds
- Maple syrup or honey (optional)

Dinner: Tuscan Tuna Tomato Pasta

- 1 package of buckwheat soba noodles or Barilla Plus pasta of choice
- 2 cans stewed tomatoes
- Olive oil
- Fresh garlic
- 1 can tuna
- 1 jar green olives
- Dry oregano
- Salt and Pepper to taste

Citrus Sea Scallops

- Garlic
- Sea scallops
- Pancetta (optional)
- Lemon
- Parsley
- Broccolini
- Cauliflower
- Olive oil
- 4 lb. spaghetti squash
- 1 lb. boneless, skinless chicken breasts, trimmed and cut into 1/2-inch-thick strips

162

- 1 Bosc pear

- Dried sage

- Fresh chives

- Fresh Parmesan flakes (Optional)

Dessert:

Apple Crisp Delight

- 6 apples

- Oatmeal (rolled oats- not steel cut)

- 1/2 cup sliced almonds

- Nutmeg

- Unsalted pasture-raised butter

- 5 pounds McIntosh Apples (or any apple you prefer)

- 1 orange

- 1 lemon

- Nutmeg

- Coconut flakes

- Ground cinnamon

- Sliced almonds (¾ c)

- Buckwheat, coconut, or spelt flour (1 cup)

- Coconut sugar or brown sugar

- Sea salt

Chapter 22

Day 22: Secret Mind Tricks to Portion Control

Why Willpower Isn't Enough

Many people are certain that if they can just muster enough
willpower, eventually misbehaving tendencies will be whipped
into docile submission. But as you know after learning about
decision fatigue, small daily decisions and temptations will
inevitably overthrow even the noblest attempts at willpower.

It is our habits, not our willpower, that allow us to accomplish
the really great stuff in life. To tame that wild animal in your
head, you have to trick it into habit autopilot.
The only way to truly overcome the seductive allure of Netflix
procrastination, sleep 'til noon sloth, or total cupcake gluttony,
is to engineer a lifestyle that will make accomplishing your
habits easy.

These habits can even be a simple as waking up at the same time, making your bed, and other ridiculously minor routines will help your brain stay focused and clear on what it is supposed to do.

So what does this have to do with weight loss and eating healthy? Everything. Understanding the science behind overeating and mastering portion control will help you build a lifestyle that makes weight loss fun and easy.

Counting calories is a great idea, but almost impossible to do with complete accuracy. Even if you are religious about it, you will find yourself deeply pontificating what exactly is an 'ounce' of cheese or a 'gram' of teriyaki sauce.

The mind-tricks below will help you shave a few hundred calories off your eating rituals. The best part is you won't even notice they're missing.

"Handy" Tricks to Dividing Your Plate

Humans have a difficult time perceiving how much we eat. One study in particulate revealed the harsh reality of human memory flaws: five minutes after eating at an Italian restaurant, 31 percent of people couldn't remember how much bread they ate, and 12 percent of people didn't even remember eating bread at all.

The best thing we can do to keep ourselves in check, is measure our food beforehand (AND tell the waiter not to bring bread). When plating your food, divide the plate in half. Fill half of it with vegetables. Then divide the second part of your plate again, and fill half of it with protein, and the other half with complex carbohydrates.

The handy guide below will loyally see you through any free-for-all buffet. These are the portion sizes in which you should consume protein, carbohydrates, and fat.

- 3 Ounces of Lean Meat = Size of Your Palm (or deck of cards)
- 1 Cup Complex Carbs = Size of a Fist (or two golf balls)
- 1 Ounces (2 Tablespoons) of healthy fats = Size of Your Thumb

Know this: If you decide to skip plating your food, drink milk from the carton, or munch on chips right out of the bag, you will unintentionally consume twice as much.

In the book "Mindless Eating: Why We Eat More Than We Think" food researcher and PhD Brian Wasink discusses multiple experiments that shed light on why people are prone to overeat without clear portion limits.

In one study, researchers gave two study groups 1/2 pound or 1-pound bags of M&Ms to eat while watching TV. Those given the 1-pound bag ate nearly twice as much. When two groups were given 34- or 17-ounce bowls and told to help themselves to ice cream, those with the bigger bowl dished out 31 percent more.

The principle of these studies makes sense: the more food is in front of us, the more of it we will eat. Buying small plates to trick yourself into eating less is a perfect example of how you can make habits that will do the work for you.

The Traceability Factor- Why Eating Buffalo Wings is an Awesome Idea

Another fascinating study by Wansink shows how the 'traceability' of food can provoke us to eat better. In this study, two groups were given unlimited plates of chicken wings to eat during a football game. One group had their bone-filled dishes cleared right away by the server, while the other test group had their plates left on the table.

The participants able to see and measure food remnants ate an average of two chicken wings less. Eating food that leaves a 'trace', like nut shells, chicken bone wings, or chocolate wrappers, will unconsciously discourage you from overeating, while giving you direct visual clues to help you better track and monitor your food intake.

Food Halos

In his book, Wansink coins the term 'Food Halos' to describe the angelic glow that brands like Whole Foods or Subway gain by being perceived as 'healthy'.

This 'halo' is dangerous because it disarms customers from making practical eating decisions. When a restaurant or brand has a 'health halo', people incorrectly assume anything they order is healthy, or that their healthy entree choice has earned them a few extra indulgences. Beware this trap.

Wansink cites a fascinating experiment demonstrating that consumers, who eat fast food branded as "healthy" such as Subway, were likely to underestimate their calorie intake by an average of 151 calories.

Customers eating at the "healthy" food chain also had a tendency to order sides, drinks, and desserts if their entrée was perceived to be healthier. These extra add-ons totaled up to 131% more calories than the entree itself.

In comparison, the customers dining at restaurants condemned for being greasy or calorie-rich ordered cautiously, in attempt to not gorge in excess on potential calorie bombs. In a similar study, people eating 'low-fat' granola consumed 21 percent more calories than those who were munching the regular stuff.

While it is probably a better idea to eat a Subway spinach salad over a Big Mac, it is also important to see what you're eating clearly, without idealistic branding clouding your vision.

Focus on Your Food

Studies show it takes about 20 minutes for the feeling of fullness from the stomach to be registered by the brain. Unfortunately, the typical fast food meal is finished in around 11 minutes.

This is why starting a meal with a salad appetizer or soup is such a clever idea. Try to savor a meal for at least twenty minutes to allow that feeling of fullness to catch up to you. TV also distracts you from how much you're eating. The more you watch, the more you're likely to eat.

In a study comparing how much popcorn viewers ate during either a half-hour show or an hour-long show, those who watched more television consumed 28 percent more popcorn.

The Power of Peer Pressure

Another interesting finding from Wansink's studies, is our tendency to mirror the habits of eating partners. If we sit with a speed-eater during a meal, we will scarf down our food. When paired with a leisurely dining partner, we begin to take our time.

That friend who is always last at the table or carting home leftovers after a meal? Invite them over sometime. Chances are, their healthy slow eating habits will rub off on you.

DINNER: Tuscan Tuna Tomato Pasta

Prep Time: 5 Minutes

Total Time: 20 Minutes

Ingredients:

- 1 can tuna
- 1-2 cans stewed tomatoes
- 1 package buckwheat soba noodles
- 2 cloves chopped garlic
- 2 tablespoons olive oil
- ½ cup green pimiento olives
- 2 teaspoons oregano
- ½ teaspoon of salt
- ½ teaspoon pepper

1. In 1 large pot, boil 2-3 cups water for pasta. Once the water is at a rolling boil, add 1 package of buckwheat soba noodles. Once pasta is soft with a slight bite, drain and rinse. *Optional:*

Season lightly with oil, salt, pepper, and garlic powder for

flavor.

2. In another large pot, heat 2 tablespoons olive oil over medium heat. Once it shimmers, add 2 cloves chopped garlic. Sauté for 30 seconds, don't let the garlic brown.

3. Add 2 cans stewed tomatoes, and let them cook. Use a spatula or wooden spoon to break down the tomatoes as they heat up.

4. Once the tomatoes are simmering, add 2 cans of tuna and ½ cup green pimiento olives. Let cook for about 10 minutes, or until warmed through. Add 2 teaspoons Oregano. Mix in ½ teaspoon of salt and pepper to taste.

5. Combine the pasta and sauce and serve.

Chapter 23

Day 23: How Eating More Will Help You Lose Weight

Your body doesn't know you live five minutes away from a grocery store and several fast food chains. It thinks you live out in a forest with a tribe, foraging for berries and hunting wild boars.

When you eat, it stores food as fat, thinking it will need it for the winter when harvest is low and boars are hibernating. Eating several small meals a day will trick your body into keeping your digestive system going all day, so it doesn't go into starvation mode and start hoarding fat reserves.

Don't starve yourself for hours to only eat so much that you feel sick or stuffed. Frequent, small snacks will protect you from getting ravenous hunger pains, followed by guilt binging.

Today's mission might be your favorite mission of all: **eat 7 meals.**

Here is your perfect daily eating routine:

7am: Protein shake

8am: Breakfast

10am: Morning snack

12pm: Lunch

3pm: *Afternoon snack

*Eat most of your carbohydrates before 4pm. If you must snack at night, eat protein snacks.

6pm: Dinner

9pm: Protein snack (if needed)

DESSERT: Amazing Paleo Apple Crisp Recipe

This recipe is gluten-free, has no refined sugar, and is reduced-carb.

Prep Time: 20 minutes

Cook Time: 45 minutes

Ingredients:

174

- 5 pounds McIntosh Apples (or any apple you prefer)
- Grated zest of 1 orange
- Grated zest of 1 lemon
- 2 tablespoons freshly squeezed orange juice
- 2 tablespoons freshly squeezed lemon juice
- 2 teaspoons ground cinnamon
- 1-teaspoon ground nutmeg

For the topping:

- ¾ c sliced almonds
- ¾ c buckwheat flour (or sub out coconut or spelt flour)
- 1/2 cup coconut sugar **
- 1/2-teaspoon sea salt
- ¾ c organic coconut flakes
- 1/2 pound cold pasture-raised butter, diced

To make a lower sugar recipe, you can cut the coconut sugar by half and add in a couple of stevia packets

Instructions:

1. Preheat the oven to 350 degrees F.

2. Butter an oval baking dish (9 by 14 by 2-inch).

3. Peel, core, and cut the apples into large wedges. Combine the apples with the zests, juices, and spices. Pour into the dish.

4. To make the topping, combine the flour, coconut sugar, salt, coconut flakes, mix thoroughly. Add in the cold pasture-raised butter in the bowl with the dry ingredients.

5. Using a pastry cutter (or your hands as a last resort), mash and cut the butter into the dry ingredients for several minutes, until you have pieces the size of peas. Scatter the topping evenly over the apples. Optional healthy/tasty addition: Add some pecan pieces mixed into the topping.

6. Place the crisp on a sheet pan and bake for 40-45 minutes until the top is brown and the apples are bubbly. Serve warm. Serve with a dollop of Greek Yogurt.

Chapter 24

Day 24: Adult Milkshakes and Diet Killers in a Can

Do you want to hear an easy weight-loss short cut? This might surprise you- it has nothing to do with what you eat. It's about what you drink. Quitting drinking your calories is so easy to do, and the weight loss benefits are worth it.

Here's why: your stomach isn't smart enough to detect liquids as calories. When you eat solid food, your stomach feels full, and you will naturally compensate by reducing your calorie intake for the rest of the day.

But if you drink liquid calories, your stomach will still crave a day's worth of solid food. If you've been reading this far, you're already avoiding milk. And soda, as you know, is diet-killer in a can.

If you're considering a trendy juice cleanse, question the nutritional benefits of milking sugar water out of fruit, only to throw away important fibrous nutrients.

Smoothie Bars like Jamba Juice are caloric traps because 'smoothies' are often over-sized ice cream bombs disguised with a health-food mustache. If you can't quit juice and smoothies, stick with nutrient-rich protein shakes, featuring vitamins, fibrous veggies like kale and carrots, hold the sorbet.

And let's be real; lattes are basically milk shakes for adults. Have you ever read the calorie count next to those drinks? It a large cup of milk, spiked with corn syrup and caffeine.

If black coffee is just too bitter for you, try an almond milk cappuccino instead. This beverage choice is high in protein, minus the dairy allergens and calories. Consider topping your drink with a sprinkle of metabolism-boosting cinnamon.

Another excellent coffee shop safe zone is the infamous superhero of weight loss: green tea. Green tea has been shown to increase fat burning and boost the metabolic rate, is filled with cancer-fighting antioxidants, and is shown to reduce risk of diseases like diabetes.

Of course, there are exceptions to every rule. There is one bizarre and fantastic drink that actually will actually cause you to lose weight. Grapefruit juice is a magical weight loss drink that has been shown to induce lower fasting blood sugar levels, better insulin sensitivity, and <u>lower levels of triglycerides</u>.

In a recent study, mice were fed a high-fat diet supplemented with small portions of clarified, pulp-free grapefruit juice. These mice gained 18 percent less weight than the water-drinking control group.

If you find yourself confused navigating the calorie-laden beverage world, included is a handy little cheat sheet for you to follow.

BREAKFAST:
If you're not a morning person, make this delicious breakfast right before you go to bed and let it sit overnight.

Banana Bread Overnight Oats

Ingredients

- 1 medium banana
- 1/3-cup oats (certified gluten-free if necessary)
- 1/4-cup Greek yogurt
- 1/2 cup unsweetened almond milk
- 1-tablespoon chia seeds
- 1/2-teaspoon ground cinnamon
- 1-tablespoon pecans
- Optional: Maple syrup or honey for sweetness

Directions

1. Mash half of the banana in a jar, container, or bowl. Next, add the oats, yogurt, milk, chia seeds, cinnamon and stir to combine.

2. Refrigerate overnight.

3. The next morning, top with pecans and the remaining 1/2 banana and enjoy.

Chapter 25

Day 25: Take the "Water Test"

Next time you're about to eat- think for a second: Are you really hungry? Or is that a thirst pang you're feeling?

It is incredibly easy to mistake thirst for hunger. You may think you are hungry, when you are actually just dehydrated. Drinking water consistently will prevent this mistake. Make hydration a regular habit will also help your body flush out toxins during your detox process.

Studies show that drinking lots of clean water, or enjoying water-based soup before meals, will cause you to eat less and make better eating decisions. The Institute of Medicine recommends men that drink 120 ounces and women 90 ounces of fluid per day. If you're active, remember to also hydrate often to replace the water you lose through sweat.

Throughout the 20 POUNDS IN 90 DAYS program, you should be drinking a little more water than usual. Here is an excellent four-part strategy for making sure your body stays hydrated.

1.) Every morning when you wake up, drink a tall glass of warm water with lemon. Eight hours of sleep with no water will make you thirsty. Adding a big glass of water to your morning routine will help cleanse and restart your digestive system for optimal functioning.

2.) Drink a tall glass (8-16 ounces) of water every 60 minutes. Schedule water breaks by putting reminders in your calendar or phone if you need to.

3.) Carry a water bottle everywhere, or keep bottles of water around the house in plain sight. You can even purchase a gallon jug of water and try to drink almost all of it throughout the day, to ensure you meet your recommended daily water intake.

4.) Take the water test. Drink a full 8-ounce glass of water and wait 10 minutes. Were you really hungry, or was it just dehydration getting to you?

Chapter 26

Day 26: Amish Hour and the Animal Alphabet

Don't you love clocking nine dreamy hours of uninterrupted sleep? Waking up feels as though you've taken a long, cool drink of water. It's great to start the day with a clear mind and rested body.

Compare that to the mornings when your bloodshot eyes click open to a panic-inducing alarm blare. You desperately wrestle for the snooze button and ponder, "Didn't my head just hit the pillow?"

Getting Zzzs is so important because hormones are regulated while you sleep, and people who get lots of regular sleep tend to make better food choices and have slimmer waistlines. You'll probably notice that the less sleep you get, the more your body craves fried carbs or decadent comfort food as an extra energy boost to get you through the day.

Sleep is a great way for you to get energy without consuming food. It also sounds simple, but the more time you spend sleeping, the less time you spend eating. Enough yammering about why sleep is incredible. We all know it's incredible. I bet you want to know, how do you get more of it?

1.) Kill the Lights

You know those nights when you burn the midnight oil, blearily staring into a computer screen, snacking, fidgeting with your phone, or watching movies? Studies have shown that light, especially blue light, suppresses our body's melatonin cycles, and undermines our effort to get in really restful REM cycles.

Unfortunately, modern technology makes it difficult to take the light out of our lives. My toothbrush has a light; my laptop charger has a light. Let's not even get started on TVs, VCRs, cable boxes, and printers. It's the 21st century, and everything has a light.

But I have a solution: grab a box of Band-Aids or some electrical tape and cover up every single one of them. Invest in some blackout curtains, earplugs, maybe an eye mask, and make your room a quiet, dark palace of sleep bliss. It's a small sacrifice that will improve your restfulness and protect your circadian rhythms.

And of course, stop looking at screens an hour before bed. In the tech industry, a new tradition called 'Amish Hour' is starting to trend. The practice is to forgo all modern electronics in exchange for reading, meditating, or hands-on creative projects right before bed.

If your iPhone doubles as an alarm clock, you'll want to set your wakeup time <u>before</u> Amish Hour starts, instead of the moment right before you crawl under your sheets.

And, for those of you who can't unplug, there is a wonderful app called <u>flux</u> that will dim your computer and iPhone based on the cycle of the sun. While you're working on getting your sleep schedule regulated, remember to get outside each day to expose yourself to sunlight to properly set your circadian rhythms.

2.) Exercise More

Maybe it's almost too obvious but, sometimes you're not getting enough sleep because you're just not tired enough. Desk jobs may be mentally exhausting, but don't give your body the physical exertion it needs.

Sometimes good old' fashioned, unrelenting exhaustion is the key to get the deep sleep you need. Do the FitQuick 9-Minute Exercise routine three times in a row followed by a 30-minute run, to burn off excess energy and sleep more deeply, guaranteed.

3.) Try the Army Crawl

If you find yourself tossing and turning the moment you hit the hay, assume this army position: rest on your stomach and spoon your mattress. Lying on your stomach with one arm and one leg out in an 'L' position will still your body. When you can't toss and turn, your mind settles itself so you can fall right to sleep.

4.) The Animal Alphabet

Counting sheep? For me it goes like this:

186

"One sheep, two sheep, three...man, sheep are so cute. That YouTube video with those alpacas set to Star Wars music is the most epically funny thing I've ever seen. I need to share that with Liz. OH NO- was it Liz's birthday this week? I think it was. Did I totally forget to get her a gift? . . ."

And then I pull out my phone to post an Alpaca video birthday message on Liz's Facebook wall. My circadian rhythms are shot to hell and the endless cycle of insomnia perpetuates.

Out of pure desperation, I found a trick that works much better than counting sheep: The Animal Alphabet. If you're having trouble quieting your mind at night, go through the alphabet and try to think of an animal with a name that starts with each letter.

For example "A is for Aardvark, B is for Beagle, C is for Cougar....". You can try this with people's names, food, places, or any category you can think of. I promise you'll be out like a light before you reach Zebra.

6.) Only Consume Carbs or Alcohol Before 4pm

Have you ever enjoyed delicious spaghetti marinara, washed down with some fruity pinot noir at around 9 o'clock at night? Or knocked back a few beers in hopes it would coax your restless mind to sleep?

Passing out in a boozy carb coma can seem like a great idea at first. But afterwards, do you also recall bolting awake in a near blind panic at 2 a.m. unable to fall back asleep?
Sugary and starchy foods spike our blood sugar levels, causing restless sleep.

Our body craves starchy foods at night for energy to stay awake. Because carbohydrates give us energy spikes, they are the last thing we should ingest right before bed.

While a lot of people think alcohol is a relaxing sleep aid, it also sharply disrupts sleep homeostasis. If you've ever passed out after drinking too much, chances are you woke up feeling exhausted. This is because alcohol prevents your brain from entering the restful REM sleep you need.

If you must snack before bed, stick to protein snacks like casein whey or almond butter to keep those dream cycles going.

7.) Minerals

When all else fails, I turn to the supplements. Melatonin is a known quick fix for a chronic sleep problem. However, be warned that this stuff packs a potent punch. If I take more than a quarter of a tablet, I'm walloped with a melatonin hangover the next day.

What often works just as well, without the next day zombie coma, is a dose of magnesium or zinc right before bed. These are nutrients we are supposed to get from the soil that our veggies grow in. But because of high food demands, soil is often over over-farmed and lacking the nutrients and minerals we need.

So to recap, if you want to get a better night's sleep: match waking cycles to the sun, sleep in a dark and quiet room, eat early in the day, exercise often, avoid alcohol, carbs, and electronics at night, and take vitamins and supplements if needed.

Want to see if these suggestions actually work for you? Download the Sleep Cycle Alarm Clock on your smartphone so you can measure your sleep quality and track how many hours you clock a night.

DINNER: Citrus Sea Scallops, Broccolini, and Faux Mashed Potatoes

Faux Cauliflower Mashed Potatoes:

Ingredients

- 1 16 oz. (1 lb.) bag of frozen cauliflower
- 2 tabs Earth Balance Butter (OR real butter, goat butter, ghee, coconut oil, or olive oil. Whatever floats your boat.)
- 1/2 tsp. garlic powder
- Salt to taste

Instructions

1. In a pot boil the cauliflower until tender (meaning you can easily pierce it with a fork).
2. Strain cauliflower and add to a food processor or blender.

3. Add remaining ingredients and process until creamy and smooth. (Note: I typically add the salt after processing so I use just the perfect amount of salt.)

Note: This same technique can be used with parsnips and or other root veggies.

Broccolini:

1. Bring 1 cup water to a boil in a large pan

2. Wash and rinse broccolini in a metal calendar

3. Place broccolini over the boiling water and let steam for 5 minutes or until coloring is a little darker than bright green

4. Season with 1 tsp. olive oil, 1/2 tsp. salt, 1/2 pepper, a squeeze of lemon juice, and a few sprinkles of garlic powder (optional)

5. For extra flavor and crisp, sauté broccolini in the same pan with the scallops

Citrus Sea Scallops

Ingredients:

- 1-1.5 pounds sea scallops
- 2 tablespoons lemon juice (save any extra lemon wedges for garnish)
- 2 garlic cloves, minced

- 1/2 tsp. salt
- 1/8-tablespoon pepper
- 1 tsp. olive oil
- 2 tsps. chopped fresh parsley (set aside half to sprinkle as garnish)

Instructions:

1. Combine all the ingredients in a large bowl. Stir to coat and let chill in the fridge for anywhere from 5 to 20 minutes.

2. Heat a dash of olive oil over medium heat in a pan. Add scallops.

3. Cook scallops FOR 2 MINUTES on each side. You will know they're ready when they're white on the outside, and pearlescent on the inside.

If you're feeling extra fancy, cook a few strips of pancetta on the side. Wrap each scallop with a slice of pancetta.

Chapter 27

<u>Day 27: Don't Be "That Guy"</u>

No one wants to be "that guy" at a restaurant. You know the one. He interrogates the waiter about 'gluten-free' menu items, orders clam chowder (hold the dairy), and seems to suspect the chef is out to poison him.

One of the biggest landmines of healthy eating are social events filled with cocktails, fried appetizers, and cheese plates. Restaurant food is also laden with creams, fats, sodium, sugar and other sneaky ingredients, just waiting to botch your hard work.

Eating healthy with others is awkward sometimes, and peer pressure can be deadly. So how do you explain to a date you can't split a supersize Coke at the movies without getting an eye roll?

The good news is, having a six-pack doesn't have to mean you are sentenced to being a hermit shut-in, feasting on plain, skinless chicken by yourself for all eternity. Instead, slyly point your friends and romantic conquests in these delicious directions:

Sushi: Healthy options are easy to find at sushi restaurants, but most people fall into the 'food halo' trap of assuming all sushi is healthy, even rice-packed rolls with cream sauce, mayonnaise, and deep-fried everything.

Hold it! There is so much deliciousness to be experienced at sushi restaurants. Enjoy fresh flavors of lean fish like Hamachi Kama (a tuna collar bone delicacy), sashimi salads, or a spicy tuna avocado roll with no rice.

Remember to go light on rice and opt-in for the 'low sodium' soy sauce. You can also start your meal with a miso soup or salad to prevent overeating. Whew- you JUST dodged that bullet.

Tapas: Why did it become so trendy to eat tiny plates for $13 dollars? It's because the Spanish know how to live, napping at 4 in the afternoon and dining all day on cured meats, seafood, and veggies that are simple and well prepared. Tapas even come in small portions, which means the calorie control is already done for you.

Greek: There is a reason that a magical, remote island in Greece holds the secret to (almost) eternal life. The Greek eat fresh, organic, local vegetables farmed in rich soil, and lean meats like lamb, fish, and chicken, hummus, spinach, and a variety of other colorful, natural foods.

Go Greek for the night with lamb kebabs, hummus, or a Greek salad, which makes not only for a tasty meal, but a long life.

Indian Food is spicy, a natural appetite suppressant, and comes in a variety of lean meat dishes flavored to perfection. Enjoy dairy free masala or tandoori, chana daal (garbanzo beans), or lentil soup for a healthy carb fix. Steer clear of 'paneer' (cheese) dishes, heavy rice, cream sauces, and go light on naan-bread.

Mexican: When eating at Mexican restaurants, remember to skip the corn tortillas and dairy. You will be pleasantly surprised when you find fajitas and huevos rancheros taste just as sensational with salsa and guacamole, instead of cheese and sour cream.

Hawaiian and **Brazilian** cuisine also has an abundance of protein dishes, including menus with lots of fish and veggies. Asian restaurants don't typically have dairy on the menu, but beware noodles, rice, and heavy MSG, sugar, or sodium in the sauces.

As for movies or social gatherings, your hosts will love you when you arrive with your own bottle of dry red wine and some hummus dip. Smuggling berries, sugar-free chocolate, or sunflower seeds into the movies will save you calories and cash on over-priced concessions.

See? You can eat healthy *and* still have a life.

Dinner: Spaghetti Squash with Chicken, Pears, and Parmesan

Delicate curls of spaghetti squash are an excellent sub for traditional pasta in this chicken dish.

Hands-on time: 30 minutes

Total time: 45 minutes

INGREDIENTS:

- 3 lb. spaghetti squash, quartered and seeded
- 1 tsp. olive oil
- 1 lb. boneless, skinless chicken breasts, trimmed and cut into 1/2-inch-thick strips
- 1 Bosc pear, cored and sliced 1/4 inch thick

(TIP: To prevent sliced pear from browning, place in a bowl of cold water; drain when ready to use.)

- 1 tsp. dried sage
- 2 tbsp. minced fresh chives
- Parmesan (optional)

INSTRUCTIONS:

1. Preheat oven to 375°F. Place squash cut side up on a foil-lined, rimmed baking sheet. Add 1/4-inch water to sheet. Bake until edges are golden brown and squash is easily pierced with

the tip of a sharp knife, about 35 minutes. Set aside until just cool enough to handle.

2.   In a large nonstick skillet, heat oil on medium. Add chicken and cook for 2 minutes. Flip chicken and add pear and sage. Sauté, stirring occasionally, until chicken is cooked through, about 5 minutes. Transfer chicken, pears and pan drippings to a large bowl.

3.   With 2 forks, scrape stringy squash flesh from skin, separating into strands. Add squash flesh to bowl with chicken mixture. Add chives and toss to combine.

4. Optional: Top lightly with Parmesan cheese, for flavor

Chapter 28

Day 28: Final Milestone Diploma

WOW. I am so impressed, and you should be too. Congratulations on reaching Day 28. Now that you've developed brand new fitness and exercise habits, you'll have to keep seeing them through until you reach the 90-day mark.

Make sure to take your "after" pics today. In the spirit of writing down and tracking your goals, your last challenge is to do your final weigh-in and measurements to see how far you've come.

Remember it takes 28 days to build new habits, but at least 90 to see full results. The healthy body you want will happen sooner than you think. Stick with this plan, and I promise it won't be long before you hear someone say 'Wow- you've lost weight!'

Often losing weight isn't the hard part, it's keeping it off that's tough. Once you reach your goals, remember to keep monitoring what you eat. Of course you'll want to celebrate your success with a treat, and you should.

To keep from pinballing back to the weight that you started at, strive to be "mostly good, most of the time". You can let loose and relax on occasion. Just make sure you stick to the principles covered in this program at least 80% of the time.

I'm always here as a resource, anytime you need me. Feel free to keep the program handy so you can start it all over again anytime you feel your will power start to slip. It's up to you now.

Keep exercising, and keep eating healthy!

Sincerely,

Chloe Black

www.fitquickapp.com

P.S. If you enjoyed this book, please don't be shy and drop me a line, leave a review, or both! I love reading feedback, and reviews are the lifeblood of Kindle books, so they are always welcome and greatly appreciated.

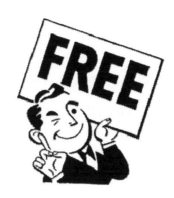

Before you devour the 20 POUNDS IN 90 DAYS Cheat Sheet, as a show of appreciation to my readers, I've put together FREE motivational resources, including a FREE exercise music playlist, 'Healthy Drinking' Cheat Sheet, and the "Before Breakfast" 9-Minute Exercise Routine.

Click HERE to receive your FREE Music Playlist, Bonus Cheat Sheet, & Exercise Plan, now!

CHEAT SHEET:

1. Set actionable, measurable goals, with a deadline
2. Write down what you want, and put it on paper
3. Make sure you set a deadline

4. Eliminate 'decision fatigue' with 'out of sight, out of mind' and throw out any junk food in your kitchen

5. Read food labels

6. Eat Colorful Foods, Avoid the White Trifecta (Dairy, Sugar, White Flour)

7. Start every morning with a dose of protein

8. Forgive yourself. If you fall off the wagon, and just keep going

9. Control your food intake with Paleo, macros, calorie counting (or all three)

10. Carbs, fat, and protein are important parts of your diet

11. Eat healthy whole grains like oats, and fats like flax oil and avocado

12. Eat (almost) as much protein as you want, and pick a healthy protein powder that works for you

13. Avoid stimulants like smoking, drugs, and alcohol

14. Break a sweat every day (9-Minute Workout Challenge), and workout at least 3 times a week, for no more than an hour

15. Start lifting heavy weights to increase your metabolism

16. Eat foods that leave a trace (chicken wings, wrapped chocolates, etc.) to discourage overeating

17. Portion your food, and don't eat straight out of the container

18. Beware health foods halos, and peer pressure

19. Enjoy a healthy snack every few hours

20. Drink water every hour

21. Avoid drinking liquid calories, except for grapefruit juice

22. Match waking cycles to the sun

23. Sleep in a dark and quiet room

24. Eat most of your carbs before 4pm

25. Avoid electronics an hour before bed

26. Go for sushi, tapas, or Greek when eating out

27. Maintenance: Be 'mostly good, most of the time'

28. Stick with it for 90 days!

FitQuickApp.com, 2015

Made in the USA
Middletown, DE
12 June 2017